Shalila Sharamon · Bodc

The
Healing Power of
Grapefruit Seed

The Practical Handbook
for Using Grapefruit Seed Extract to Heal Infections,
Allergies, and Much More
One of the Most Effective New Healing Remedies

LOTUS LIGHT
SHANGRI-LA

1st Edition 1996
2nd Edition 1997
Lotus Light Publications
P.O. Box 325
Twin Lakes, WI 53181
The Shangri-La Series is published in cooperation with
Schneelöwe Verlagsberatung, Federal Republic of Germany
©1995 by Windpferd Verlagsgesellschaft mbH, Aitrang, Germany
All rights reserved
Translated by Christine M. Grimm
Edited by Julia Kemp, Michael Tanner
Cover design by Wolfgang Jünemann,
based on an illustration by Berthold Rodd
Interior illustrations: Alois Hanslian
Total production: Schneelöwe, D-87648 Aitrang

ISBN 0-914955-27-6

Printed in the USA

...nothing in the world is as powerful
as an idea
whose time has come.

VICTOR HUGO (1802 - 1885)

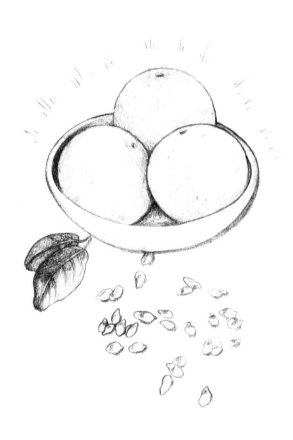

Table of Contents

The First Encounter

But where there is danger,
the possibility of rescue also grows.

FRIEDRICH HÖLDERLIN (1770 - 1843)

In our search for possibilities of natural healing, one day we came across an amazing and promising substance. In its "coded" form we had frequently encountered it before—as the seed of a common fruit. How often had we spit out the bothersome seeds of the grapefruit, unaware of the hidden treasure inside them. How this treasure was ultimately discovered and the enthusiastic response of both researchers and the people who use it will be described in the following chapter.

Other than many of the familiar natural remedies, no tradition has been handed down for grapefruit seed extract. It is a "new" substance, and research is constantly being carried out regarding its effects and scope of application. Yet, it comes in the nick of time for many "new" diseases that have become prevalent as a result of our modern lifestyle.

Our first encounter with the extract of the *Citrus Paradisi* (its botanical name) took place at a little health food store in our adopted home of Ireland. The day before, a friend had told us how her protracted intestinal complaints had been healed through grapefruit seed extract. "Grapefruit seed extract? Never heard of it." But when it smiled at us from the counter of the health food store, our curiosity was aroused. The owner had just recently become acquainted with the substance. He told us how, after years of trying other remedies in vain, grapefruit seed extract had, within weeks, cured his *Candida albicans*. With growing interest we listened to his stories about a variety of chronic complaints among his friends and customers that had been healed even more rapidly.

Then he handed us a copy of a newspaper article from England. Some of the key words describing the antibacterial effect of the grapefruit seed extract caught our eye: "Broad spectrum—powerful and effective—non-toxic—non-weakening to the immune system—little or no impact on the beneficial bacteria—inexpensive—well researched—naturally derived—hypoallergenic."

Now this really sounded wonderful. Had Mother Nature actually given us a remedy that effectively repels pathogens—without weakening the immune system, destroying the intestinal flora, and all the related consequences?

We continued to read, and soon we were totally enthusiastic. "Effective against more than thirty fungi and a host of single-cell parasites." Alarming reports on the "invasion of fungi" which can no longer be denied since the use of dark-field microscopy, came to mind. Various experts estimate that about half of all diseases can be attributed to an internal fungal infection and recent research work appears to confirm a correlation between fungi and such diverse diseases as arthritis, allergies, cardiovascular complaints, and many others.

Studies in the USA have come up with similar findings on parasites, including the news that one-quarter of New York's population is supposedly infected with them. The increasing stress in our modern civilization, an unnatural lifestyle, and today's common unhealthy diet loaded with additives have weakened our immune system to the point that it can no longer meet the challenge of defending us from the many invaders. They make themselves at home in our body, developing their hidden effects within it.

As we read about the effect of grapefruit seed extract in the little health food store, a quote from Hölderlin came to mind:

"But where there is danger, the possibility of rescue also grows."

If the extract from the seed of the *Citrus Paradisi* keeps the promise that it makes, it would certainly be an invaluable gift from "God's pharmacy" for the people of our age.

During the following weeks we put out our feelers and information about grapefruit seed extract flowed in from everywhere. Research results, data, and facts, as well as reports on experiences arrived from the USA, Canada, Korea, Peru, Mexico, Kenya, Thailand, England, Ireland, France, Denmark, and Germany. Our astonishment about its enormous scope and effectiveness grew from day to day.

However, so far, we didn't have any first-hand experiences with the extract. "Unfortunately," we were both relatively healthy. Still, we started to take a few drops every day as a test. To Shalila's surprise, she had slight symptoms of detoxification that were similar to those she had experienced while fasting. Was it possible that some invaders had slipped into her body unnoticed and were now being disposed of? In any case, after about two weeks, we felt fresher than we had in a long time. No cold has succeeded in getting a foothold with us since then. At the first sign of an itchy throat, we reached for the grapefruit seed extract and the problem vanished in no time. Although a wave of influenza caused everyone around us to cough and sneeze, we were spared.

At the same time, we recommended the extract to friends and acquaintances with corresponding symptoms and asked them to share their experiences with us. We treated our cat's dermatomycosis (fungal disease of the skin), sprayed our aphid-infested plants, watered our sprouts, and washed our hair with it, just to name a few of our many experiments. The success was so convincing that we wanted to share the "good news" with as many people as possible. The idea for this book was born.

Despite all this, it was clear to us that even the most effective remedy cannot replace the inner learning process to which an illness tries to draw our attention. Neither can it replace the change to a healthier diet and a more natural way of life. In order to achieve lasting, deep-reaching, and holistic healing, it may be inevitable that we change our inner attitudes and convictions together with the way we live, think, and eat. On the other hand, it can take a very long time before an inner transformation manifests itself in the dense matter of our body since we all know that matter is much slower than the mind.

This means that healing should start on all levels, and grapefruit seed extract can apparently play a very significant role on the physical level. The experience of a new clarity and freshness, which often accompanies the elimination of the diverse unwanted invaders, can also awaken the desire to constantly maintain and even increase this new quality of life. Ideally, it can prepare the path to a more conscious lifestyle and inner growth.

It is our wish that many people will achieve better health and an increased sense of well-being by using grapefruit seed extract in this way. We also hope that this book will stimulate further research on this very promising extract and inspire producers of remedies to include grapefruit seed extract, with its many possibilities, in their range of products. We are certain that in the near future this extract will replace a large range of synthetically manufactured medications, hygienic preparations, preservatives, and pesticides, all of which can have highly questionable side effects.

A Tree Called
"Citrus Paradisi"

Through the perfect world of the plants,
God in His infinite goodness
has given the human being
almost everything
that he needs for his food,
clothing, and healing.

JOHN GERARDE, 1636 IN HIS HERB BOOK
"THE HERBAL OR GENERAL HISTORIE OF PLANTES"

We don't know what might have inspired the botanists to give the meaningful name of *Citrus paradisi* to the grapefruit tree out of more than 60 citrus varieties. They could scarcely have suspected anything of the hidden treasure within the seed of the grapefruit since its valuable qualities have only recently been discovered. The ability of its active ingredients to free the body from so many undesirable invaders can certainly bring us a little bit closer to "paradise."

The oldest mention of the grapefruit tree comes from the 17th century when this evergreen fruit tree, ranging from 4 to 25 meters in height, was discovered by botanists on the Caribbean island of Barbados. It was assumed to be a variety of the shaddock or pomelo tree, which originates in Southeast Asia and still grows wild there today. The plant was probably named "grapefruit" because the fruit characteristically grows in bunches or clusters. The citrus plants belong to the genus of rue plants (Latin: Rutaceae). The most familiar species of these are: lemon, orange, tangerine, citron, lime, bitter orange, bergamot, shaddock, and of course the grapefruit.

The grapefruit tree has dark-green, oval, shiny leaves and develops clusters of fragrant white blossoms with five petals each. The first fruit appears after four to seven years. A mature tree gives us the enormous amount of 500 to 700 fruit a year. One fruit has a diameter of 4 to 9 inches and weighs

11

between 7 oz. and 1 lb. This means that a single grapefruit tree can bear nearly 7 cwt of fruit in one season.

In 1823, the grapefruit was first brought from Barbados to Florida, where it was cultivated commercially. More and more farmers started growing this new fruit in increasingly larger plantations. In Florida alone, where today the world's most extensive grapefruit plantations are found, more than 2.5 million tons of grapefruit are harvested annually. Large cultivation areas are also located in Spain, Morocco, Israel, Jordan, South Africa, Brazil, Mexico, Jamaica, and Southeast Asia.

Large quantities of the fruit are processed into juice. In the USA, grapefruit juice is a popular breakfast drink. In many countries the fruit is mixed into salads and enjoyed as a healthy entree for meals. Some new varieties of grapefruit have just a few or no seeds at all. This shows how little attention has so far been given to the seeds since there was no apparent use for them.

The plants, which thrive even in poor sandy soils, prefer a location just above sea level. They need an average temperature of 77 degrees F. Frost or low temperatures can seriously damage them. Growing in warm, sunny countries, the fruit store a daily sunshine dose of 7 to 8 hours. While they are ripening, their content of fruit sugar and juice increases while the level of acid decreases. Once harvested, the fruit cannot continue to ripen, but the ripe fruit stays fresh on the tree for several months and can be picked at any time.

The Components

The flesh of the round, yellowish grapefruit is primarily used for the production of fruit juice, often as an addition to other fruit juices. The juice contains the bitter-tasting glycoside naringin and is rich in vitamin C and vitamin B_1.

The main active ingredients of the fruit peel are: pinene, limonene, linalool (alcohol), and citral aldehyde, with an oil content of 21%. These components are generally recognized as anti depressive, refreshing, and stimulating for the blood circulation and the thalamus (interbrain), thereby promoting a natural activation of chemical processes. They enliven the emotions and the mind. The grapefruit peel also contains flavinoids (flovone is the Latin word for yellow plant pigment).

Flavinoids were called vitamin:P in earlier times. They are used frequently in compound preparations together with ascorbic acid, citrin, hesperidin, rutin, and quercetin. Furthermore, the substances in grapefruit peel have a generally antiseptic effect.

Dissolved in a fatty oil, these ingredients can be combined with other substances, resulting in interesting preparations such as massage oils, shower gels, and bubble bath. For 1 pound of cold pressed peel essence, more than 100 pounds of fresh fruit peels are required. In aromatherapy, grapefruit peel oil has become increasingly important today.

The **seeds** of the grapefruit contain bioflavinoids and glycosides in the form of naringin (naringenin rutinosid), isosacuranetin (didymin), neohesperidin, hesperidin, dihydrocampherol glycoside, poncirin, quercetin glycoside, campherol glycoside, apigenin rutinoside, heptamothoxyflavone, nobiletin, as well as several proteins.

There are two manufacturers who are the principal suppliers of the concentrated extract to other companies who then supply the retail market. The extract is manufactured by a bio-technical process from grapefruit seed and pulp. This is rolled and ground and then extracted with vegetable glycerine. We now know that this is not a simple extraction process but that new compounds are formed. It is therefore not clear as to whether the extract should be described as natural. It is however plant based and the early literature called it a natural product. The extract is proven to have a strong growth inhibiting effect on bacteria, fungi and some viruses coupled with extremely low toxicity for humans, animals and plants. These tests have been carried out in a number of research laboratories around the world. (The results are described in detail in the chapter on "Scientific Data and Facts". It has also been used extensively by Naturopathic Practitioners, in natural cosmetics and remedies.

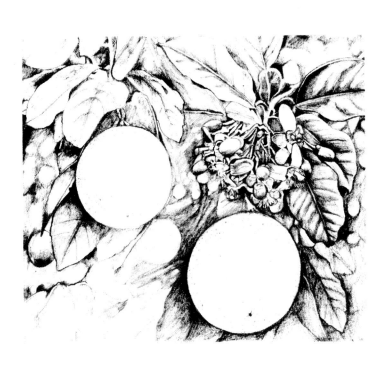

A Universal Remedy
Is Discovered

Coincidence
is necessity
shrouded in veils.

BARONESS MARIE VON EBNER-ESCHENBACH
(1830 - 1916) FROM "APHORISMS"

It happened in the year 1980 in a compost heap: An attentive hobby gardener noticed that the grapefruit seeds in his compost didn't rot. As coincidence would have it, this hobby gardener didn't just enjoy gardening, but was a physician, an Einstein Laureate physicist, and an immunologist specializing in the investigation of natural remedies. His curiosity aroused, Dr. Jacob Harich of Florida—the name of the hobby gardener—took a closer look at the phenomenon in his compost heap. The result was more than remarkable. A substance was concealed in the grapefruit seeds that appeared to be more effective, and at the same time less harmful, than any known antibiotic.

But that wasn't all. Research undertaken by a number of renowned institutes* brought to light an unexpected broad spectrum of efficacy. The extract from the seeds of the grapefruit was found to not only inactivate viruses and bacteria, but also yeasts and other fungi, as well as parasites. In comparison, the effect of conventional antibiotics is limited to bacteria alone.

1. The ideal antimicrobial should be broad spectrum since we rarely know for sure the individual germ or mix of germs. Research results show that grapefruit seed extract is effective

---

* Among them: the Pasteur Institute in France; the Institute for Microecology in Herborn, Germany; the University of Sao Paulo, Brazil; the University of San Marcos in Lima, Peru; the University of Georgia in Athens, Georgia; the Universidad Automóma de Nuevo in Monterey, Mexico; the Brigham Young University in Utah; the University of Arkansas; the University of Malaya in Malaysia; the University of Ricardo Palma, Mexico; the South American Interlab Laboratory, S.A.; the Southern Research Institute, USA; the US Department of Agriculture; and many more.

against approximately 800 bacteria and virus strains, 100 strains of fungus, as well as a great number of single-cell parasites. No other known antimicrobial can demonstrate such versatility.

2. It should be powerful and effective. Grapefruit seed extract develops its antimicrobial activity at very low concentrations. Most microbes will be killed within the range of 2 - 1000 ppm (9 drops in a liter is 100 parts per million). In addition, the previously mentioned versatility of grapefruit seed extract is clear proof of its powerful potential. In comparison to other remedies, grapefruit seed extract shows excellent results. An international research team* examined the effect of grapefruit seed extract on 770 strains of bacteria and 93 fungal strains during 1989-90 and compared them with 30 effective antibiotics and 18 antimycotica (fungicides). Grapefruit seed extract was found to perform as well as all the tested agents. Similar results were reported by the Great Smokies Laboratory in Ashville, North Carolina, a leading center for stool analysis, where grapefruit seed extract is tested routinely together with other natural and chemical antibiotics on a wide variety of germ cultures. In these studies also the results for grapefruit seed extract were outstanding.

3. The ideal antimicrobial should be non-toxic. In this respect we would like to relate a little incident reported by Richard Starr, the president of the Bio/Chem Research Institute in Lakeport, California. In Peru, where grapefruit seed extract is used for disinfection of agricultural products, a drunken agricultural worker inadvertently drank about 3 or 4 fl. oz. of the liquid extract that some jokester had put into a whiskey bottle. Apparently this unusually high dose helped more than it hurt: the farm worker passed all kinds of worms and said he never felt better.

According to scientific research, it would take at least 4,000 times the normal dose to produce a possible life threatening effect. This means that a person weighing 180 lbs. would have to drink about 2.2 pints (American) or 1.75 pints (Imperial) of

---

* Ionescu, G./Kiehl, R./ Wichmann-Kunz, F./ Williams, Ch./Bäuml, L./ Levine, S.: "Oral Citrus Seed Extract in Atopic Eczema: *In Vitro* and *In Vivo* Studies on Intestinal Microflora," *Journal of Orthomolecular Medicine*, Volume 5, No. 3, USA, 1990.

33% liquid grapefruit seed extract (20% extractives) for it to be potentially fatal.

4. The ideal antimicrobial should be non-weakening to the immune system. This criterion is more than fulfilled. In fact, grapefruit seed extract has been used with success for a variety of immunodeficiency diseases since its broad spectrum antimicrobial activity relieves the immune system of an enormous burden.

5. The beneficial bacteria should remain intact. Initial research indicates that grapefruit seed extract, taken in a normal dose, doesn't touch the important Bifidobacteria and only insignificantly reduces the Lactobacilli, despite its inhibiting effect on harmful intestinal bacteria. In addition, it appears that the beneficial intestinal flora can thrive much better after yeasts and other pathogens have been destroyed.

6. The ideal antimicrobial should be largely naturally derived since synthetic chemicals have an unpredictable short- or long-term effect on the body. Grapefruit is a gift of nature in all its parts. The extract is made by grinding the seeds together with a portion of the flesh membrane, thereby fulfilling this criterion as well.

7. The ideal antimicrobial should be hypoallergenic since many of us suffer from sensitivities to customary antibiotics. Most doctors could not establish any kind of allergic reaction in the use of grapefruit seed extract. However, Dr. Allan Sachs points out that about 3 to 5 per cent of all people are allergic to citrus fruit and could therefore also display a sensitive reaction to grapefruit seed extract. These people should start with a low dosage and, when possible, use the pulverized extract with its somewhat lower acidic content in comparison to the liquid form.

Two further criteria related to cost effectiveness and adequate scientific research. Both of these points were also satisfactorily fulfilled.

After these convincing results and a fund of personal experience, Dr. Allan Sachs published a series of articles in American magazines that, along with other publications, gave rise to growing interest. More and more holistic health practitioners, doctors, and other medical professionals became aware of the new substance, that has no side effects. They then began prescribing it to their patients as an effective alternative to synthetic and mold-derived preparations.

Today there are many doctors who can look back on years of experience with grapefruit seed extract. The most frequent applications lie in the area of gastrointestinal diseases, yeast infections, colds, throat- nose- and ear-infections, fungal diseases of the nails and skin, gum inflammations (gingivitis), and vaginal infections, to name but a few. An important application is in the support of the immune system and protection against infections for patients with chronic immunodeficiency symptoms like AIDS, chronic fatigue, or Candida. New applications are constantly being discovered.

Doctors who have an adequate amount of experience with grapefruit seed extract are overwhelmingly positive in their evaluation. They appreciate the extract not just because of its incredible range of application and its effectiveness, even where other remedies fail, but also because it is very well tolerated by their patients.

"There's something unique about this particular substance. Whatever it does, it does it without debilitating side effects. It has the advantage of being very safe." This statement comes from the internist Dr. Leo Galland of New York who has prescribed the extract for the past seven years and has published various reports about its effect on *Candida*. Dr. Louis Parish, M.D., an investigator for the US Department of Health and the FDA, who treated many people suffering from intestinal diseases, is also full of praise: "Grapefruit seed extract gives more symptomatic relief than any other treatment."

The pediatrician and health correspondent of the popular American television program "Home Show," Dr. Jay N. Gordon of California, emphasizes its high efficiency in dealing with the frequent yeast infections in both the mouth and diaper area of his smallest patients, which are often difficult to cure. In a letter to one of the manufacturers of grapefruit seed extract, he praises its complete non-toxicity: "You have an excellent, extremely safe formulation that I have found to be completely safe for even the very youngest babies in my practice." The German physician Dr. Klaus Küstermann, M.D., of Baden-Baden, who has treated many of his patients with grapefruit seed extract, discovered that: "In my opinion, grapefruit seed extract is absolutely the best, most effective antibiotic and fungicide that nature has given us."

We also met with extraordinary enthusiasm from *users* of grapefruit seed extract. They were often astonished at how quickly their symptoms disappeared, how a few drops of the extract in a glass of water could stop diarrhea or the flu, how eczema, skin fungus, dandruff, warts, and sweaty feet simply vanished. Many of them could hardly believe it when their chronic vaginal or intestinal *Candida* or their many years of gum disease finally healed after no other remedy had brought lasting success. Others came to value grapefruit seed extract as an indispensable travel companion that helped against food poisoning and cholera, as well as small wounds. Meanwhile in some family medicine chests, the extract has become a trusted remedy and a valued friend.

Despite all this, it appears that the potential of grapefruit seed extract has still not been fully exploited. Research continues at various institutes, such as the Pasteur Institute in France, one of the leading European institutes in the research of AIDS, where the extract's efficacy against the HIV virus is examined. Further tests and studies are currently in progress in Canada, Denmark, Germany, and Korea. General recognition is gradually growing on a broader basis. For example, in Austria the substance is widely recognized as the product of choice against *Candida*, and in Mexico it is a commonly accepted remedy for various diarrhea diseases.

Yet, the possibilities for using grapefruit seed extract are not limited to the area of human medicine alone. Animals profit equally from this highly effective and safe antimicrobial. Organic farmers in Denmark have used the extract for their animals with excellent results. In large farms for pigs, cattle, and poultry, as well as in horse-breeding, it has been possible to drastically reduce cases of disease and death by adding the pulverized grapefruit seed extract to the feed. (Although we think "factory farming" is undesirable as a matter of principle, we still want to mention these results. All of the farms concerned used grapefruit seed extract within the scope of a holistic, healthy way of feeding and keeping the animals.)

A farmer from Denmark reported that of the 30 piglets born every year on his farm only 16 survived. The rest died of PRRS (Porcine Reproductive Respiratory Syndrome). The vet didn't know how to help. After the farmer introduced the extract, not a single piglet died anymore. Another farmer was advised to butcher his cows that suffered from mastitis. With the help of grape seed extract, the mastitis was healed overnight, and the cows were soon back to their normal milk production.

A further encouraging example for the use of the extract in animals was reported from Peru. For many years, the high death rate among the alpacas due to various infectious diseases had been a cause for concern. Vaccinations and antibiotics had not provided any reliable results. In an experiment with grapefruit seed extract, carried out by Dr. Guillermo Calderon, Professor for Immunology at the University of San Marcos in Lima, Peru, a solution to the problem was finally in sight. The mortality rate of these graceful animals, which provide us with the softest and finest type of wool, was reduced from 50% to 2%.

Fish can also benefit from the special qualities of grapefruit seed extract. In Chile, the zoologist Dr. Carlos Roman tested the extract as a remedy against the oxygen-stealing algae infestation in salmon tanks. While the tanks remained free of algae, he did not notice any kind of toxic effect on the fish. Quite the opposite! In low concentrations, grapefruit seed extract also promotes good health in fish.

Many people who have learned to value the beneficial effects of grapefruit seed extract for themselves have also tried it on their pets. Pet-owners were thrilled to report that they had finally found an effective and healthy alternative to the customary chemical vermifuges (anti-worm agents). Fungal diseases in animals were just as effectively healed as those in human beings, and some bothersome vermin apparently no longer felt as happy in fur sprayed with grapefruit seed extract. Lovers of aquarium fish were glad to now be able to keep the water in the aquarium free of algae in a simple and non-toxic way.

Yet, the possible uses of grapefruit seed extract go still beyond the application for people and animals. In Central America and South America, where the warm temperatures permit bacteria and mold to quickly destroy agricultural produce, the extract has been widely adopted as an effective and inexpensive mold- and spoilage-inhibiting agent. It is used for grains, fruits, and vegetables, as well as for disinfecting and preserving fish and meat. A test left no doubts about the efficiency of grapefruit seed extract as a preservative: the shelf life of fruits and vegetables could be increased three to four times. Organic farmers in Denmark apply the extract as a natural based pesticide for potatoes, leeks, and carrots.

The cosmetic industry was also quick to respond to the extremely successful test results on the versatile, germ-killing properties of this extract. A non-toxic, odorless preservative was exactly what many manufacturers were looking for in order to keep their products free from chemicals. The chemicals that are usually used for preservation are often toxic and can interfere with the activity of some of the herbal constituents. Grapefruit seed extract appears not only to perform remarkably as a preservative, it even seems to enhance the activity of many herbal products.

The extract has also gained entrance to many homes as a safe disinfectant and is particularly welcome where small children live. A few drops added to diverse household cleaners, dishwashing soap, or laundry detergents ensure a germ-free environment.

In the USA, the germ-killing properties of grapefruit seed extract are also valued in many hospitals, where it is used in the cleaning of bed linen and carpets—the most popular dwelling places for bacteria, fungi, and other pathogens. Jerry Skidmore, manager of Laundry Operations for the "Florida Hospital" wrote: "I have had 30 years experience in the laundry industry and it is only since using it (*grapefruit seed extract*) that I have had the peace of mind and assurance that the people in our hospital and the other hospitals we serve have a complete protection from fungal and bacterial infections that can be associated with linen. It is very gratifying to know that even after many hours of exposure to the various bacteria that are always present in hospitals that our linen has been tested and found free of all harmful or pathogenic organisms." In higher concentrations, grapefruit seed extract is used for sterilizing and disinfecting operating rooms, as well as medical equipment such as inhalers.

A great cause for concern in many hospitals is the resistance to the usual disinfectants by an increasing number of pathogens. Here as well, grapefruit seed extract offers an effective and completely non-toxic alternative.

In addition, grapefruit seed extract renders excellent service in disinfecting the skin as a post-operative measure. In contrast to the common agents, it attacks only the bacteria and not the skin. Dr. J.A. Botine of the University of Sao Paulo, Brazil, reported that the extract was 100% effective as a disinfectant compared to 98% effectiveness for the usual agent and only 72% for alcohol.

A further promising possibility for the use of grapefruit seed extract is in the treatment of drinking water. Many countries, cities, and communities are looking for less expensive and more progressive and healthy methods of treating sewage water. Today we know that long-term damage cannot be ruled out by using chlorine for this purpose. Sensitive intestinal flora can be damaged by chlorinated water, for example. In addition, various pathogenic micro-organisms like *Giardia lamblia* have become resistant to chlorine.

In two independent tests, carried out by the microbiologist John R. Carson and the Armadillo Environmental Service in the USA, it was found that grapefruit seed extract is particularly suited for sewage-water treatment. At a dilution of approx. 350 liters of grapefruit seed extract in 1 million liters of water, the count of fecal coliform bacteria was consistently reduced to less than 1 per 100 ml; a count of 200 per 100 ml is generally accepted as adequate disinfection. If we add the lack of toxicity to this effectiveness, we have an ideal, environmentally friendly agent for treating sewage water.

In 1994, the Danish expert Knud Dencker-Jensen was commissioned by his government to develop a practicable concept for biological treatment of drinking-water within the scope of a development-aid project in Thailand. He used grapefruit seed extract for this purpose—with excellent results. We hope that such projects will soon be copied in many countries.

In South America, grapefruit seed extract has been used for quite a long time in lieu of chlorine in a variety of public swimming and bathing applications, particularly where light clouding of the water by the extract is of no significance. If exceptional water clarity must be maintained, often a portion of the chlorine is replaced by grapefruit seed extract. Many private owners of whirlpools or swimming pools already enjoy chlorine-free—and therefore healthy and odorless—bathing pleasures, thanks to the miracle in the seed of the grapefruit.

Last but not least, the quick, biological degradability should be mentioned. Results of a five-year study in the USA with repeated experiments in which solutions of different strengths were sprayed over the soil showed a complete decomposition of grapefruit seed extract after one to eight days. The extract was then recognized in the USA as being "non-ecotoxic." Wonderful!

Grapefruit Seed Extract for External Use

There is a large range of symptoms for which grapefruit seed extract can be applied externally. Wherever bacteria, viruses, fungi, or other parasites have caused diseases of the skin or mucous membranes, the extract can create the preconditions for healing by killing the pathogens. Freed from the undesired micro-organisms, the body can carry out the healing process without any difficulty. If you would like to do even more, you can support the regeneration of the skin and mucous membranes through *aloe vera*, for example.

A great wealth of experience is available when it comes to the external use of grapefruit seed extract. Holistic health practitioners and doctors who prescribe the extract for their patients report extraordinarily good healing success.

Grapefruit seed extract should generally not be used in full strength. We have made special mention of the few exceptions to this rule. For some applications, it is advisable to dilute the extract with oil instead of water. Almond, olive, sesame, or avocado oil are particularly suitable for this purpose. The extract should always be mixed well with the water or the oil. Never let grapefruit seed extract get into the eyes since it can cause strong irritations. *In case of an emergency, immediately wash out the eyes with lots of warm water and consult a physician, if necessary.*

When using ready-made grapefruit seed extract products, please always pay attention to the instructions for use and the dosage information on the package.* In case of doubt, ask a doctor, pharmacist, or therapist for advice.

---

* **Please note:** The dosages given in the following chapters relate to the normal retail strength usually labelled as 33%. This dilution is one part of a proprietory grapefruit extractive (which is itself 60% grapefruit extractives and 40% glycerine veg. U.S.P. since glycerine is used in the extractive process), to which 2 parts of glycerine or water have been added. This dilution therefore contains only 20% portion of grapefruit extractives, since the basic extract already contains 40% glycerine. A declaration of 20% extract would therefore be more correct and companies are encouraged to declare the actual strength.) Where very large amounts are used and our figures relate to the undiluted, 60% basic extract, we mention this clearly in the text. We have suggested, that all producers offer the same strengths and drop size in order to avoid confusion with dosages. **You should always check the strength and dosage instructions on the bottle.** The dosages in the book are based on a drop size of 30 drops = 1 ml.

Mouth and Lips

Antiseptic Mouthwash
Grapefruit seed extract is considered an ideal mouthwash with a strong antiseptic effect. Harmful bacteria and germs are eliminated and reinfection is delayed. Gargle thoroughly three times daily with 5 drops of extract in a glass of water. The mouthwash will leave your breath fresh for a long time.

Mouth ulcer
Aphtae are painful little ulcers of the mucous membrane in the mouth, created by the reactivated herpes virus. Rinse out the mouth several times daily with 10 drops of grapefruit seed extract in a glass of water. In addition, dab the mouth ulcer with 2 drops in a tablespoon of water using a cotton swab.

Ulcerative Stomatitis
Put about 10 drops of grapefruit seed extract in a glass of lukewarm water, mix well, and rinse out the mouth and gargle with it several times a day. The grapefruit seed extract will promote healthy gums and fresh breath at the same time.

Thrush (Fungal Infection of the Mouth Region)
Thrush appears as a whitish coating in the mouth and is caused by the yeast fungus *Candida albicans*. Thoroughly rinse the mouth about 3 times daily with 5 to 10 drops of grapefruit seed extract in a glass of water. The less bitter powder is recommended for children. Open a capsule and mix half of the powder in a glass of water. If necessary, add some fruit juice to improve the taste. The fungus likes to settle on pacifiers and nipples of baby bottles, leading to constant reinfection. To; disinfect, put them into a solution of 20 drops in 1 liter (35 fl. oz.) of water for about 20 minutes. Rinse very well before using them again.

Bad Breath
Bad breath can be caused by bacteria inside the mouth, tooth decay, or putrefaction in the lower digestive tract.
Rinse the mouth and gargle with 5 to 10 drops of grapefruit seed extract in a glass of water several times a day. This will

keep your breath fresh for quite a while. If the cause is in the digestive tract then you should also take the extract internally.

Cracked Lips
Dilute a few drops of grapefruit seed extract with a tablespoon of oil and apply several times a day. Grapefruit seed toothpaste, available commercially, has proved successful for treatment. It also contains calendula and glycerine and is applied directly to the lips. Grapefruit seed extract ointment is also suitable for this purpose.

Sunburn or Glacial Sunburn on the Lips
To prevent infections, apply a mixture of several drops of grapefruit seed extract in one tablespoon of oil twice daily. The ointment available commercially has also proved successful.

Cold Sores (Herpes Simplex)
Blisters on the lips occur due to a reactivation of dormant herpes viruses. Apply a mixture of several drops of grapefruit seed extract with one tablespoon of oil 2 to 3 times daily to the affected spots using a swab. Let the preparation take effect overnight. Use again as soon as there are any signs of blisters forming again.

Teeth and Gums

Plaque
Plaque is a bacterial coating of the teeth that is considered to be the cause of dental caries and periodontosis. Put 1 to 2 drops of grapefruit seed extract on the moistened toothbrush and extensively brush the teeth 3 times a day. The grapefruit seed extract toothpaste available commercially can also be used for this purpose. Additionally put 5 to 10 drops of grapefruit seed extract into the water you use to rinse after brushing your teeth. To clean the spaces between the teeth, soak dental floss with grapefruit seed extract or put some drops into your "water pik." Grapefruit seed extract can be very effective in preventing plaque.

Caries (Tooth Decay)

Caries is a demineralization process of the tooth enamel and the hard substance of the tooth, caused by the metabolic processes of plaque bacteria. Use the same treatment as described under "Plaque."

Toothaches

Gargle several times a day with 10 drops of extract in a glass of water. In addition, a cotton pad soaked in 3 drops mixed with an egg-cup of water can be placed directly on the aching tooth.

Tooth Extraction

We recommend that you gargle with a solution of 10 drops of grapefruit seed extract in a glass of water. This can prevent wound infection and relieve the pain.

Gum Inflammation (Gingivitis)

Inflammation of the gums, often accompanied by bleeding, is caused by plaque bacteria. Their metabolic products have the effect of a cellular poison that attacks the gums. Grapefruit seed extract has proven to be very effective in dealing with this problem. The bleeding often disappears after just a short time. For treatment, put 1 to 2 drops of grapefruit seed extract on the moistened toothbrush and thoroughly brush the teeth 3 times a day. When rinsing after brushing, add 5 to 10 drops to the water. It is also advisable to add it to your "water pik." For severe complaints, you can put a few drops of the extract mixed with an egg-cup of water on a moist strip of cotton wool and place it on the gums for several minutes every day.

Toothbrush Cleaner

The toothbrush very often houses the same bacteria that cause us problems within the mouth. They find a welcome breeding ground in the moisture between the bristles. Grapefruit seed extract is excellently suited for killing undesirable germs and thereby preventing possible reinfection. Put 10 drops of extract into a glass of water, mix well, and place the toothbrush into it for about 15 minutes or even leave it there overnight. Rinse well before using it again in order to remove the dead germs. *The water in the glass should be changed every few days.*

Nose and Paranasal Sinuses

Nose Rinse
Put about 3 drops of grapefruit seed extract in an egg-cup of lukewarm water and mix well. Using a pipette, drip a few drops of the mixture into both nostrils while leaning your head back. Move your head from side to side and back and forth, sniff in several times and then strongly snort out. *Do not drip undiluted extract into the nose.*

Runny Nose (Rhinitis)
Dab the inside of the nose with a solution of 3 drops of grapefruit seed extract in an egg-cup of water using a cotton swab several times a day. If available, spray grapefruit seed extract nasal spray into the nose 3 times daily. As a further measure, grapefruit seed extract should be used internally.

Nasal Ulcer
Using a solution of 3 drops of grapefruit seed extract in an egg-cup of water, swab the affected region several times every day with a cotton swab.

Sinusitis
Do a nasal rinse (see above) several times a day or use a grapefruit seed extract nasal spray. In addition, the extract should also be used internally.

Throat Area

Sore Throat/Tonsilitis
Put 10 drops of grapefruit seed extract into a glass of luke-warm water and gargle extensively with the solution 5 to 6 times a day. In addition, the extract should also be used internally.

Coughs
Gargle several times a day with 10 drops of grapefruit seed extract in a glass of lukewarm water. If commercially available, grapefruit seed extract cough medication like sprays or

lozenges can be used as well. In addition, the extract should be used internally.

Hoarseness
Gargle 3 times a day with a solution made of 10 drops of grapefruit seed extract in a glass of lukewarm water. It is particularly recommended that you use a product that also contains glycerine. Many singers (for example, Mick Jagger—we've heard) use glycerine to keep their vocal chords smooth.

Laryngitis
Use as above: Put about 10 drops of grapefruit seed extract into a glass of lukewarm water and gargle with it 3 times a day.

Ears

Ear Cleaning
Mix 10 drops of grapefruit seed extract well with an egg-cup of glycerine or oil. Drip several drops of this mixture into the ears 1 to 2 times a day. *Never put the extract in its undiluted form into the ears!*

Earaches
Application as under "Ear Cleaning." The commercially available grapefruit seed extract ear drops can also be used.

Inflammation of the Middle Ear (Otitis Media)
Use as under "Ear Cleaning". The commercially available grapefruit seed extract ear drops can also be used. In addition, the extract should be used internally.

Face

Acne/Spots/Pimples
Moisten the face, rub about 5 drops of grapefruit seed extract into the moist hands, and thoroughly massage into the face. Let it take effect, wash off well, and dab dry. A light tingling of the

skin may occur, indicating that the skin has been thoroughly cleansed. If the extract gets into your eyes, wash out very thoroughly with water. A grapefruit seed extract skin cleanser is also advisable. The extract has a lasting antiseptic effect.

Shaving
Several drops of grapefruit seed extract added to the shaving lather guarantees immediate antiseptic care of wounds when even the smallest injuries occur during a wet shave. The extract can also be put onto the blade directly. In a diluted form, it may be an interesting addition to aftershave.

Scalp and Hair

Treatment Shampoo
Put a portion of shampoo into your hand and mix 5 to 10 drops of grapefruit seed extract into it. Massage into hair and scalp for about 2 minutes. Rinse out well afterwards. For eczema or undefined skin irritations on the scalp, the extract can also be used as a lotion. To do this, soak a cotton pad in a solution of 20 drops of grapefruit seed extract in an egg-cup of water and dab the scalp with it. If the extract gets into the eyes, immediately wash out thoroughly with water.

Dandruff
Dandruff is often caused by a fungus of the scalp. Treat as described under "Treatment Shampoo." Use the shampoo and/or lotion about 2 to 3 times a week, later once a week. After the formation of dandruff has diminished, continue the treatment every two weeks as a preventative measure.

Itching Scalp
If possible, the cause should first be clarified. Try treating it according to the directions under "Treatment Shampoo" and observe the reaction. If successful, repeat the application.

Head Lice
Head lice are increasingly widespread. We were very successful with a mixture of one-third grapefruit seed extract and

two-thirds shampoo. (If you wish, you can experiment with a smaller dose.) Mix well and spread evenly over the entire scalp and hair. Cover the hair with plastic and allow the extract to take effect for 20 to 30 minutes. Repeat after 3 days.

Skin

As an Emergency Remedy
Grapefruit seed extract has proved to be an ideal emergency remedy for smaller injuries, burns, and other problems. Whether for small accidents while on trips, during sports, at work, or in the household—the extract with its helpful, antiseptic effect can be used everywhere. Grapefruit seed extract should always be in any backpack, first-aid box, bag, and in any family or company medicine chest.

Smaller Cuts, Skin Abrasions, and Scratches
All smaller injuries and burns can be given antiseptic care with grapefruit seed extract. Best suited for this purpose is the commercially available grapefruit seed extract skin spray, sometimes also called "First-Aid Spray." If this is not on hand, dilute several drops of extract with some water and put it carefully on the wound.

Minor Burns
Cover with grapefruit seed extract ointment or skin spray. Never apply the full-strength extract.

Rashes
For non-specific rashes, try to first clarify the cause. However, even if this isn't possible, grapefruit seed extract offers good chances of improvement. Mix 10 drops of the extract with oil and apply to the skin. Ready-made ointments, as well as the skin spray that is commercially available, can also be used. Apply 2 to 3 times a day and observe the effect. If there is an improvement, continue the treatment until the symptoms have subsided.

Dermatitis

First of all, don't wash with soap. After washing the affected skin areas, rub in a mixture of 10 drops of extract in an egg-cup of oil. A grapefruit seed extract ointment containing moisture, if possible, can also be used for this purpose.

Psoriasis

Put 10 drops of grapefruit seed extract into an egg-cup of oil and apply to the affected areas of skin twice daily. Observe the reaction, and continue to use if there is an improvement.

Shingles (Herpes Zoster)

Use as described under "Psoriasis."

Eczema

For dry eczema, mix 10 drops of grapefruit seed extract with an egg-cup of oil and apply. Lotions or ointments with grapefruit seed extract are equally good for application. If the affected surfaces are very small, a drop of undiluted extract can also be applied. For weeping eczema, grapefruit seed extract powder should be used. (It has only been commercially available as foot powder up to now.) The extract has proved to be extremely successful for eczema.

Nettle Rash

Many people have had good experiences with grapefruit seed extract for nettle rash as well. Apply the usual mixture of 10 drops of extract into an egg-cup of oil to the itching areas of the skin. Skin spray can be just as beneficial.

Insect Bites and Stings

Apply grapefruit seed extract in an undiluted form. If the skin is sensitive, mix with a bit of water or oil.

Tick and Leech Bites

Drip the grapefruit seed extract directly onto the tick or the leech, then remove and put another drop of extract on the bite itself.

Ulcers of the Legs / Varicose Ulcers

Soak a clean compress or wound pad with a mixture of 30 drops of grapefruit seed extract and an egg-cup of boiled (and cooled) water and place on the affected region. Renew repeatedly.

Warts
The removal of warts may require some patience, but grapefruit seed extract has proved to be quite effective in many cases. Put a few drops of the undiluted extract on the warts twice daily on a regular basis.

Skin Fungi
Fungal diseases of the skin can be quite difficult to eliminate, but grapefruit seed extract has proved to be very successful for the various types of fungal skin diseases due to its excellent fungicidal effect. We have heard of various cases where people have rubbed the undiluted extract onto the affected spots, but it can also be mixed with some glycerine. Use twice daily on a regular basis. The treatment should be continued for some time after symptoms have disappeared since the skin fungus often has not died completely and could grow again. Expose the skin to a great deal of fresh air and sunshine.

Feet

Athlete's Foot (Mycosis Pedis)
Because of the special conditions on the foot, such as a relatively constant level of moisture, darkness, and warmth, a fungus can grow here particularly well. Athlete's foot can be very stubborn, but many cases have demonstrated that even the most resistant foot fungus can be eliminated over time by the highly fungicidal effect of grapefruit seed extract. If the afflicted regions are not too sensitive, the extract is frequently applied in full-strength. Otherwise, it can be diluted with glycerine. If "weeping" occurs, use grapefruit seed extract foot powder, which also has proved effective for the prevention of athlete's foot. Furthermore, about 20 drops of grapefruit seed extract should be added to the last rinse when washing socks or stockings in order to avoid reinfection. The inside of shoes can be treated with powder. Always dry the feet well after bathing or showering. Sunshine is also helpful against fungi.

Sweaty Feet

Sweaty feet are also caused by fungi. Foot powder or foot baths with grapefruit seed extract have proved effective for this problem. Add about 50 drops to a foot bath for this purpose. After soaking the feet, dry them well. For prevention of reinfection, the same measures apply as described under "Athlete's Foot."

Callouses (Horny Skin)

A warm foot bath lasting 5 to 10 minutes with 30 drops of grapefruit seed extract is very helpful in facilitating the removal of the horny skin and is a good disinfectant for the feet at the same time.

Corns

Put one drop of grapefruit seed extract undiluted on the corn once or twice a day.

Thorn and Sting Warts

Once a week, file off the callous spots using a coarse file or sandpaper or carefully cut or scratch them off with a sharp knife (scalpel). Use some old newspaper to catch the pieces in order to prevent the spread of infection. Then apply one drop of grapefruit seed extract twice daily. Continue to apply the extract for several weeks after the symptoms have disappeared. The removal of these warts is usually a very lengthy matter. Regular use of grapefruit seed extract as a foot powder or as an addition to soap or the foot bath has a good preventative effect.

Blisters

Apply 1 to 2 drops of grapefruit seed extract on the blisters for disinfection purposes.

Fingernails and Toenails

Nail Fungi

Fungal diseases of the nails are usually very difficult to heal. They develop extremely slowly and gradually spread to the adjoining toenails or fingernails. People afflicted by this disease hardly notice it getting worse, but the appearance is deceptive. Over the years, or even decades, the fungus will grow deeper and deeper into the nail bed. Furthermore, it can be transmitted to other people. Action should be taken as soon as possible, that is to say at the first visible sign of a change in the nail.

Grapefruit seed extract has proved very effective against this difficult disease. Before application, the affected nail should be filed down as far as possible over a newspaper catching the filing dust, using a coarse file or sandpaper. (To avoid transmitting the fungus to other nails, the file should be disinfected with grapefruit seed extract after use and the newspaper with the filing dust thrown away.)

After this has been done, apply the extract twice daily in an undiluted form. The affected area of the nails should be filed again every 3 to 4 days, later every 3 to 4 weeks. Continue to apply grapefruit seed extract twice daily. It is very important to keep up this routine for several months. The effort is worthwhile since complete healing can only be attained through persistence, which also applies to the use of chemical agents against nail fungus. (If you have ever seen—or even smelled—a nail fungus in an advanced stage, you will spare no effort to cure it.)

For preventative purposes, the regular use of grapefruit seed extract as an addition to liquid soap or hand cream, foot powder, or a foot bath is advisable. If the toenails are affected, add about 20 drops of grapefruit seed extract to the last rinse when washing socks or stockings and spray the inside of the shoes with grapefruit seed extract spray to prevent reinfection.

Cuticular Infections

This infectious disorder often begins inconspicuously, yet it can quickly develop into an extremely painful condition that continues for weeks. Frequently only a surgeon can help in the end—unless you have the helpful grapefruit seed extract to hand and immediately massage a few drops into the affected groove of the nail bed 2 to 3 times daily. The infection usually subsides very quickly thanks to the antibacterial effect of this extract. An effective treatment requiring very little effort! A warm finger bath in water or oil with a few drops of grapefruit seed extract can also provide relief.

Vagina and Genitals

Vaginitis

Vaginitis can be caused by bacteria, fungi, or parasites. Don't wash the vaginal area with soap, but add a few drops of grapefruit seed extract, possibly together with tea tree oil, to the water you use for washing. Use the following vaginal rinse for at least one week: Add 1 to 3 drops of grapefruit seed extract to a 6 to 8 fl. oz. glass of warm water and mix well. (If desired, 5 drops of echinacea tincture can also be added.) Draw this mixture into a commercially available syringe (without the needle), carefully insert, and squirt the mixture into the vagina. To do this, lie on your back and lift your pelvis. Instead of a syringe, a feminine douche that you can buy in pharmacies may also be used. Repeat every 12 hours during the first 3 days of the treatment, then once a day.

A further possibility is to soak a tampon with the prepared mixture and insert for between 1 to 6 hours (depending on what feels right for you). The grapefruit seed extract can be mixed with sesame oil instead of water, which has an additional beneficial effect on the mucous membranes and protects them from drying out. About 20 drops of grapefruit seed extract can be added to the last rinse when you wash your underwear in order to avoid reinfection.

In addition, panty liners can be sprayed with a grapefruit seed extract skin spray. To regenerate the vaginal flora after the treatment, mix some natural, unflavored yoghurt with an equal amount of warm water and squirt it into the vagina. The success rate for treatment is extraordinarily good.

Never use the seed extract in its undiluted form in the vaginal area!

Fungal Infections of the Vagina (Yeast Infections)

If the vaginal infection has been caused by a fungus (*Candida albicans*), the measures described above should be applied and even continued for some time after the symptoms have disappeared. The sexual partner should always be informed in the case of a fungal infection since he will usually be affected as well. (See "Fungal and Parasitic Diseases in the Male Genital Area.") In most cases of a *Candida* infection in the vagina, the intestines are infected by the same yeast fungus. It is therefore advisable to treat the intestines at the same time. (For more information, see the chapter "Grapefruit Seed Extract for Internal Use.")

Vaginal Parasites

One of the most frequent types of vaginal infections is caused by a microscopic parasite by the name of *Trichomonas vaginalis*. The infestation becomes apparent through a putrid-smelling vaginal discharge with inflammation and burning in the vagina. It is estimated that about 30% of all women are affected by this parasite at some time. It is usually transmitted by sexual intercourse and can cause a non-specific urethritis (inflammation of the urethral mucous membrane). See treatment instructions under "Vaginitis."

Feminine Hygiene

Grapefruit seed extract can also be used for general hygiene in the vaginal area. Add a few drops to the water you use for washing. A grapefruit seed shower gel which contains no soap or a skin cleanser containing grapefruit seed extract can be used as well. *Never use the extract in its undiluted form in the vaginal area!*

Fungal and Parasitic Diseases in the Male Genital Area

Fungal and parasitic infections can be transmitted very easily during sexual intercourse. For this reason, the male partner should also be aware of the possibility of being infected. A few drops of grapefruit seed extract can be spread onto wet hands and rubbed into the penis for treatment purposes. Don't rinse it off afterwards. A mixture containing 10 drops of extract in an egg-cup of sesame oil is also suitable for this purpose. Let it take effect for several minutes. *Grapefruit seed extract should never be poured onto the penis in its undiluted form* since this could lead to intensive irritation.

The measures outlined above should be continued for about 2 weeks. The chances of being cured are very good. In addition, add 20 drops of grapefruit seed extract to the last rinse when washing your underwear for the next several weeks in order to prevent reinfection. Grapefruit seed extract soap, shower gel, or skin cleanser can also be used as a preventative measure. If the infection has spread to the urethral mucous membrane, it is advisable to also take the extract orally. Please refer to the instructions for internal use.

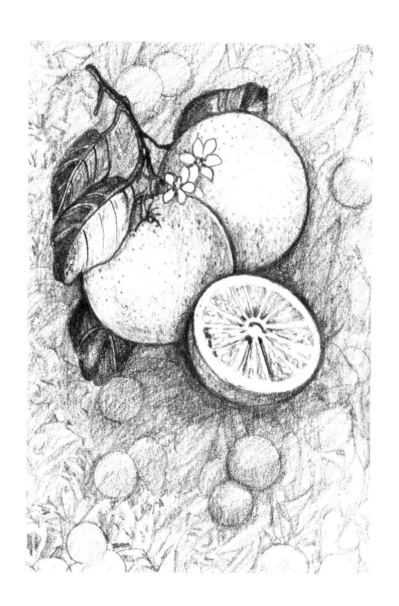

Grapefruit Seed Extract
for Internal Use

It is general knowledge today that bacteria and viruses cause a great many internal diseases or participate in their development. The enormous extent to which this also applies to fungi and parasites is only now being gradually recognized. The symptoms that occur through an infection with fungi or parasites are frequently identical to those of a bacterial or viral infection. This gives rise to false diagnoses time and again, resulting in ineffective treatment. To our knowledge, grapefruit seed extract is the first remedy that covers various types of micro-organisms at the same time. The list of lab analyses in the appendix of this book indicates the extremely large spectrum of pathogens for which this extract is effective.

The knowledge about the healing effects of grapefruit seed extract has entered into an increasing number of practices working with naturopathy. As a result, a great fund of experience has become available to us, particularly in the area of external applications, gastrointestinal diseases, and colds, which have become the main areas of use. Yet, reports by various doctors and health practitioners, as well as experiences with animals, indicate a clear effect of grapefruit seed extract also beyond these specific areas throughout the entire body. However, little or no research has been carried out on the living organism regarding the many diseases whose pathogens have been destroyed in the lab tests.

In the following survey of the internal use of grapefruit seed extract, we have tried to limit ourselves to those diseases and health disorders that have been adequately documented. We hope that this book will stimulate further research and that we will soon be able to report on new results. We are convinced that grapefruit seed extract can in the near future become a healthy alternative, without side effects, to antibiotics and synthetic preparations.

Grapefruit seed extract combines very well with other natural remedies. It is a great team player and seems to augment the activity of other medicinal herbs. Homeopaths particularly value it because is does not interfere with the activity of homeopathic remedies.

However, beyond the great help it can provide, grapefruit seed extract is most beneficial as part of a holistic health program. It should not become a quick substitute or a makeshift solution replacing a necessary change in our eating and living habits. Our illness might be telling us something about our life situation, and we shouldn't try to avoid its message. When inflammations recur in the same or other places, even after repeated use of grapefruit seed extract, we should ask ourselves why this is happening and think about any reorientation that might be necessary.

Phlogogenic (inflammation-causing) micro-organisms prefer to settle in those areas of the body where they come across weakened tissue. This weakening is frequently caused by toxins that have settled in the body. Environmental poisons, additives or residue in foods, as well as mercury amalgam fillings in the teeth, are the most frequent source of poisons that enter our body from the outside world. These are joined by poisons from within. Processes of decomposition and putrefaction caused by unbalanced nutrition and deficient digestion, metabolic waste products, and toxins produced by micro-organisms are the sources of inner poisoning.

These poisons can hardly gain a foothold in the body as long as the life in us continues "to flow." Only when the flow of energy in one area of our body stagnates is the ground prepared for the invasion of toxins and pathogens. The reversal of this process is used by treatments such as acupuncture, for example, which stimulates the energy flow in the affected area of the body and can often eliminate the symptoms through this measure alone.

Blocks in the flow of life energy are created by stress, tensions, fears, negative expectations, and similar problems. The mental and emotional background of health disorders comes into play here, which sets the stage for its physical expression. Every area of the body symbolizes a certain mental or emotional ability. For example, the heart shows the ability to feel and both give and receive love, our legs represent the ability to advance in life, our digestion shows us how well we can "digest" experiences, and our immune system symbolizes our ability to remain authentic and defend ourselves against harmful influences. With the help of our body's symbolic language, an illness or functional weakness in a certain area of the body can tell us which ability has become blocked or lost.

If we want to eliminate illness in a fundamental and lasting manner, we should start on the different levels. Measures on the mental and emotional level such as relaxation, letting go of fears, and accepting our deeper needs should be accompanied by cleansing and purifying the body from toxins, avoiding repeated poisoning, and freeing the body from damaging micro-organisms.

Within such a holistic healing program, grapefruit seed extract can support the healing process on the physical level in a wonderful way.

Instructions for Internal Use: For internal treatment, we usually take 3 to 15 drops of grapefruit seed extract 2 to 3 times daily in a full glass of water or a corresponding number of capsules or tablets until the symptoms have disappeared. (The packages usually contain information on how many drops correspond to a capsule or tablet.) The drops are dissolved in glycerine and should be thoroughly mixed with the water. If the taste is too bitter, you can alternatively take the extract mixed in a glass of fruit juice. The powder contained in the capsules is usually less bitter. This makes it particularly suitable for children. You can open a capsule and mix its content or part of its content into a glass of water. A more precise dosage is possible in this manner.

It is advisable to start with a small dose and slowly increase it. There are a number of reasons for this. The most important one is the so-called "die-off" reaction. When bacteria, fungi, or other pathogens begin to die, toxins are set free, possibly leading to some discomfort or tiredness.

However, according to our experience, a distinct reaction of this type usually occurs only in the first treatment with grapefruit seed extract or when there are greater intervals of time between treatments. Apparently, together with the pathogen of the acute disease, a great number of other pathogenic micro-organisms, which have settled unnoticed in our body, are largely disposed of with the first treatment. If such reactions occur, it is normally recommended that you decrease the dose or keep it low and increase it very slowly. We have had very good experiences with the additional ingestion of psyllium husks. These husks come from the seeds of "Indian fleawort," a grain-like panicle plant (*Plantago ovata* and *isphagula*) and have the quality of absorbing several hundred times their own weight in fluids. They clean out the digestive system by absorbing toxins and waste substances together with the fluids in the intestines, enabling them to be excreted.

Psyllium husks are packaged loose in pharmacies or drug stores or sold as powder in capsules. About 1/2 oz. of the seeds (= 3 teaspoons) can be taken 2 to 3 times daily mixed into a glass of water. Because the husks swell rapidly, drink the mixture quickly and rinse it down with more water. Ready-made preparations should be taken according to the manufacturer's instructions. (Do not use in cases of intestinal obstruction, unstable diabetes, or pathological constriction of the esophagus or gastrointestinal tract.) In addition, it is very important to drink large amounts of pure non-carbonated water in order to support de-toxification by flushing the kidneys. Water from the tap containing chlorine should be "de-chlorinated" by boiling it without a lid for 30 minutes.

It is advisable to take a pro-biotic such as live culture yoghurt to help restore the friendly bacterial flora which is damaged in most people. Take 1 part live yoghurt mixed with 2 parts of warm water, daily, some hours apart from taking the grapefruit seed extract. As already mentioned, about 3 to 5% of the population are allergic to citrus fruits and can therefore also show a greater sensitivity towards grapefruit seed extract. If you suffer from an allergy to citrus fruits, start with a dose of 1 drop of extract in a glass of water and slowly increase it in accordance with your reaction. You can also try taking the less acidic powder.

We have realized that people with a sensitive stomach sometimes react with a slight feeling of resistance. This can be avoided by taking the extract *after* meals or eating a snack before taking it. The stomach usually adjusts to the new remedy very quickly, and you can then take it independent of meals. However, in such a case it is also best to start with a dose of a few drops and slowly increase it.

For a repeated intake of grapefruit seed extract, you can usually start with a dose of 6 to 8 drops. However, all dosage descriptions are just general guidelines that may vary in individual cases. Always pay attention to the information on the package inserts.

We would like to emphasize that a doctor, naturopath, or holistic health practitioner should be consulted in the case of serious or lasting health disorders or diseases. We hope that grapefruit seed extract will find its place in more and more practices and—where appropriate—will be available as the remedy of choice, so that a growing number of diseases can be healed in an alternative way under competent supervision.

Inflammations in General

Most diseases are accompanied by an inflammatory process. Inflammations are a reaction of our immune system to influences that damage or destroy cells and tissue and thereby obstruct the normal functioning of our body. Among these influences are various types of micro-organisms like bacteria, viruses, fungi, and parasites. Further influences are toxins that either enter the body from the outside or are produced by micro-organisms found within the body. The body's own processes like metabolism or fermentation and decomposition of food can also produce toxins that burden the body in a similar way. Another main group is formed by the nutrients that are seen as harmful by the body and treated accordingly (see under "Allergies") because of the body's inability to deal with them. If the immune resistance is weak, various micro-organisms that normally lead a harmless existence in the body can also become pathogenic and lead to illness.

The various invaders are usually repulsed or inactivated by our immune system. Toxins are neutralized by the so-called antitoxins or detoxified by the liver. If the resistance is successful, the **inflammation** caused by the micro-organisms or toxins will subside.

However, it appears that the natural immune resistance is increasingly incapable of protecting people in our modern age.

The overloading with environmental poisons, the increasing stress of our modern way of life, rushed meals and unbalanced nutrition, as well as antibiotics, appear to strain or weaken our immune system. When a lack of immune resistance is combined with additional overloading of the liver through toxins, various poisons are deposited in the organs and tissue. Germs can then make themselves at home in our body over a long time producing **chronic inflammations**.

Today we are faced with the situation that, thanks to modern achievements, the great epidemics that afflicted our ancestors have been largely eradicated, but we are increasingly plagued by chronic diseases. Although serious illnesses are less frequent, many people are never completely healthy. At the same time, diseases associated with a weakening of the immune system, such as **cancer** or **allergies**, have gradually turned into the modern "plagues."

With the active ingredients in the seed of the grapefruit, nature has given us a remedy in our time of need that can enormously relieve our immune system. As already mentioned, grapefruit seed extract has proved its efficacy for approx. 800 strains of bacteria and approx. 100 strains of fungi. In addition, there have been very good experiences with the elimination of parasites. Even if the effectiveness of the extract for some of the diseases whose pathogens were destroyed in the lab tests has not been adequately researched on the living organism, both **acute** and **chronic inflammations** can improve in many cases through the general relief provided for the immune system.

As an additional benefit, micro-organisms like parasites or fungi, very often overlooked as the cause of an illness and therefore not treated, can be destroyed due to the broad spectrum of efficacy of grapefruit seed extract even when they haven't been diagnosed.

As mentioned above, inflammations can also be caused by toxins. Grapefruit seed extract can't free us directly from these poisonous substances. It can, however, help decrease the toxic strain by killing those micro-organisms that release toxins within the body. The liver and immune system can then concentrate on the other poisons and dispose of them more effectively.

The "poison-producers" among the micro-organisms are frequently located in the intestines, and we have a great deal of experience available from the many successful applications.

44

Elimination of the harmful pathogens in the intestinal area is the precondition for reinstating the natural ecology of the intestines. When the intestinal flora is healthy, it is difficult for bacteria, fungi, and parasites to settle and/or spread and cause damage to the body.

We therefore think that grapefruit seed extract can be effectively used, in at least a supportive manner, for every type of inflammation including chronic inflammations that indicate a weakening of the immune system.

Dosage: 3 to 15 drops 2 to 3 times daily in accordance with the "Instructions for Internal Use."

Colds

Flu infections and **true influenza** are among illnesses classified as colds. Both types are produced by viruses. **Flu infections** are **acute disorders of the respiratory tract**, usually accompanied by **fever**. They manifest themselves in a **runny nose, hoarseness, coughing, sore throat, headache** and **pain in the limbs**, as well as **exhaustion. Dizziness, tachycardia, bronchitis,** or **diarrhea** can also occur.

True influenza usually develops in a similar manner, but it is more severe than the **flu infection**. It is caused by the *influenza viruses of the types A, B, and C.* World-wide epidemics (pandemics), which occur at irregular intervals, are triggered solely by the *type A* virus. In between the world-wide pandemics, epidemics occur in individual countries at intervals of about two to three years. *Variations of the respective A virus* from the last pandemic are responsible for these epidemics.

In a laboratory test with the *influenza A2 virus*, it was possible to prove the efficacy of grapefruit seed extract even for this extremely virulent (aggressive) form of pathogen. Many people report quick relief or healing of their "**cold**" with the practical application of grapefruit seed extract.

Apart from the various *external* applications (see the chapter on "Grapefruit Seed Extract for External Use"), it is recommended that grapefruit seed extract be taken internally. A very good combination is echinacea and grapefruit seed extract.

Dosage: 3 - 15 drops 2 to 3 times daily in accordance with the "Instructions for Internal Use."

Gastrointestinal Infections

Various pathogens, which usually get into our body through contaminated food or water, can produce an **infection of the gastrointestinal tract**. This manifests itself in **diarrhea**, often accompanied by **pains in the stomach, nausea**, and **vomiting**. Among the most frequent pathogens are *coli bacteria (Escherichia coli)*, *salmonella*, and the poison from *staphylococcus*. A **viral infection of the gastrointestinal tract** can also occur, primarily in the cold seasons. Severe infectious diseases like **bacillary dysentery** (caused by *Shigella flexneri, sonnei*, and *dysenteriae*), **amebic dysentery** (caused by *Entamoeba histolytica*), **cholera** (caused by *Vibrio cholerae*, a rod-shaped bacillus that lives in water), as well as typhoid fever and **paratyphoid fever** (caused by *Salmonella typhi* and *paratyphi*), are less common and occur almost exclusively in southern latitudes.

Grapefruit seed extract appears to develop an excellent effect in the gastrointestinal tract. Doctors who worked with the extract recorded a high degree of success with the various **gastrointestinal infections**. Many people report that the outbreak of the illness can be avoided if the extract is taken at the first sign of a **gastrointestinal infection**.

According to the experiences of various experts, a great many people in whom **colitis** or **Crohn's disease** is diagnosed, a disease whose cause seems unknown, are actually infected with *Shigella, Salmonella*, amoebas, fungi, *Giardia lamblia*, or other parasites. Frequently there is also a mixture of these various pathogens. With the elimination of the pathogens, the symptoms usually disappeared.

We have also heard of various cases where the serious infections mentioned above were successfully treated. Dr. Louis

Parish, doctor and investigator of the American Department of Health and the FDA, has used grapefruit seed extract within an experimental program and treated about 200 patients suffering from **intestinal problems**, including **dysentery**, with great success. According to him, grapefruit seed extract brought greater symptomatic relief than any other treatment.

In laboratory tests, the extract has proved a high level of efficacy for all pathogens of severe infections (see list of laboratory analyses in the Appendix). More extensive research on the practical applicability of grapefruit seed extract for this area would be worthwhile. People living in southern countries, in which these diseases are still prevalent, could profit enormously from an inexpensive remedy.

In warm countries, such as in Africa and India, there are occasionally large cholera epidemics with many deaths. In Europe, the last great cholera epidemic occurred in Italy in 1973. The use of grapefruit seed extract to treat patients, as well as disinfect contaminated drinking water, could contribute to saving many human lives in the case of a cholera epidemic.

We recommend people who travel in southern countries to take a few drops of extract every day for prevention. See the chapter "The Smallest Portable Medicine Chest in the World."

Dosage: In case of illness, take 3 - 15 drops 2 to 3 times a day in accordance with the "Instructions for Internal Use." If there is suspicion of severe infection, take the extract according to the directions of a doctor or naturopath.

Gastritis, Gastric and Duodenal Ulcers

In 1979, the American pathologist Robert Warren discovered a bacterium, *Helicobacter pylori*, that nests in the stomach lining and damages the cells. Bacteria are normally destroyed by stomach acid. However, *Helicobacter* has an alkaline "mantle" that protects it from the attack of stomach acid. Once this bacterium has settled in the mucous coat of the stomach, it reduces the production of protective mucous, exposing the stomach and upper digestive tract to the acidic digestive juices. In this way it promotes the development of **gastritis, inflammations,** and **ulceration.**

A young Australian doctor, Barry Marshall, conducted a research project on *Helicobacter* together with Robert Warren in the year 1984. They discovered that the great majority of patients with an inflamed or ulcerated stomach was infected with this bacterium. Today we know that the risk of duodenal ulcers is increased up to five times if *Helicobacter* is present. At least 95% of the patients with **duodenal ulcers** are housing *Helicobacter.* **Digestive complaints, heartburn, dyspepsia*,** and many other gastrointestinal disorders improve once this bacterium is eliminated.

Researchers from Stanford University reported in the Journal of the National Cancer Institute that almost all patients with the most common type of **stomach cancer** are infected with Helicobacter.

Infection with *Helicobacter* can also lead to a series of consecutive symptoms. Because the balance of acids and enzymes is disturbed and digestion is impaired, **toxicity** and **food intolerance** increase. The intestinal flora suffers and **inflammatory, infectious,** and **allergic diseases in the intestines and the entire body** are promoted. According to Dr. Mendall of the British Heart Foundation, chronic inflammation caused by *Helicobacter* can even set up **coronary heart disease.** The probability of developing **cancer** is increased six-fold, as the above-mentioned Stanford University researchers report. In some cases, the slowly growing cancer "MALT-lymphoma" was healed through elimination of *Helicobacter.* However, for most cancer patients, it is not enough to kill the bacterium alone since too much damage has already been done. The main medical debate today is to what degree cancer can be prevented by eliminating *Helicobacter.*

A large number of people are unknowingly infected with *Helicobacter.* According to a study in England, no less than 20% of the twenty-year-olds, 40% of the forty-year-olds, and 60% of the sixty-year-olds are infected. The reduction of stomach acid and decrease in immunity, which often accompany the ageing process, appear to promote infection with *Helicobacter.*

---

* A less severe form of an acute nutritional disturbance in infancy.

Grapefruit seed extract helps us in dealing with this undesirable bacterium as well. In laboratory tests, the extract killed Helicobacter at a concentration of 1 : 1000.

Dosage: 3 - 15 drops 2 to 3 times a day in accordance with the "Instructions for Internal Use." As a maintenance dose, it is recommended that you take 10 - 15 drops in a glass of water half-an-hour before meals on an empty stomach 2 to 3 times a day until the symptoms have disappeared.

Candida Albicans
and Other Fungal Diseases

"Fungi are just as important as bacteria and viruses in causing disease." This explosive assertion is propounded by the Swiss naturopathic doctor and researcher Bruno Haefeli, who has dedicated his work to the research of fungal diseases (mycosis). Naturopaths and health practitioners estimate that more than half of their patients are afflicted with fungal diseases. Just ten years ago, fungal diseases of the intestines and inner organs were an exception.

Mycosis is a symptom of our modern lifestyle. The basic precondition for a fungal disease is an impaired immune system. Antibiotics and cortisone, stress, inundation with environmental poisons, unbalanced or inferior nutrition, food additives, etc., all weaken our immune system or disturb the natural symbiosis within our body. This then prepares the ground for the multiplication of fungi.

Experts consider the various types of mold and yeast fungi to play an important role in the development of such different diseases as **cardiovascular complaints, rheumatism, arthritis, gout, asthma, allergies, sinusitis, gastritis, tuberculosis, cancer,** and many more.

The mold fungus *Mucor*, for example, attacks the **red and white blood cells** and causes **circulatory disturbances**, among other things. *Aspergillus*, a further mold fungus, prefers to settle in the **lymphatic system** and **joints**, and the mold fungus *Penicillium* is involved in **inflammations**.

49

In addition, mold fungi produce some of the strongest poisons we know. The best-known is probably *Aflatoxin*, which often occurs in peanuts and Brazil nuts, as well as in a large number of other foods. One hefty dose of this poison can debilitate parts of the liver for a long time, possibly for years. Mold fungi can be found in humid areas in nature, in damp rooms, or on the soil of house plants. Foods like bread or other dough products (above all, when they are packaged in plastic), cheese, jam, and fruit juices can all be infested by mold fungi, even before they are visible. They don't spare fruit, vegetables, or salad either. Furthermore, mold fungi are increasingly used by the food industry for processing foods. With their help, for example, flour is made light and fluffy, instant potatoes are "peeled," fruits intended for making juice are "pre-mashed," and the taste of meat is improved.

Fungi gain entrance to our body when we inhale and eat food. If they meet with a lack of resistance, they can invade and spread.

Mold fungi are joined by yeast fungi. The best-known, most frequent, and most damaging among them is *Candida albicans*, which can affect the entire body. Microbiologists and fungus researchers have discovered 25 different varieties of this yeast fungus in the human body. According to experts, up to one-third of the population of the industrialized nations suffers from diseases associated with *Candida albicans*. *Candida* usually grows in the intestines without causing any damage. But if our natural defenses are poor, this harmless fungus can overgrow, spread throughout the intestines and penetrate into inner organs such as lungs, kidneys, or heart. Our skin and mucous membranes can also be attacked by *Candida* (see the chapter "Grapefruit Seed Extract for External Use").

The overgrowth of Candida in the intestines and its invasion into inner organs can produce a large range of symptoms. Among these are **flatulence, diarrhea, colitis and ulcers in the digestive tract, female disorders, including sterility, fibrosis, or pregnancy problems, and male disorders, including prostatitis.** Further symptoms are **allergies, hyperactivity, hormonal imbalance, heart problems, headaches, migraines, poor memory, poor balance, earaches, asthma, sinusitis, kidney problems, fluctuations in blood-sugar levels, meningitis, and gastritis.**

The various symptoms are caused by the *poisons* of the fungus *Candida* which produces almost 100 different toxins. One of these poisons is a substance similar to a hormone that can unbalance the hormonal system. Another poison can attack the brain or nerves. Large amounts of alcohol can also be produced by *Candida*. In a company in Japan, workers were fired because they constantly showed signs of alcoholic intoxication. Although they protested that they hadn't had a drop of alcohol, tests showed a high level of blood alcohol. *Candida* was ultimately determined to be the cause of the problem.

The various poisons represent a great strain on the liver, which now can no longer adequately detoxify the body of the many other toxins that get into it. Fatigue, a general feeling of discomfort, and depression join the other symptoms.

Experts estimate that 7,000 to 12,000 people die in Germany every year of fungal infections. Yet, orthodox medicine has failed to recognize the extent of fungal diseases and few doctors assign the various symptoms produced by fungal diseases to the true cause of illness. False diagnoses are therefore a common occurrence.

It is actually not easy to diagnose a fungal disease. The fungus tests employed by orthodox medicine, such as stool analysis, do not provide any certainty. Even determination of the antibodies is unreliable since a weakened immune system often no longer produces enough antibodies.

In this situation, a special method of blood analysis is employed by various experts: In a dark-field microscope, rarely used in biology and medicine, light-rays fall in from a low angle, making otherwise invisible structures and movements in the blood visible. A different method was developed by the above-mentioned Dr. Bruno Haefeli. He uses a special staining technique to recognize fine living structures in the blood. Under the influence of light, the stained fungi suddenly grow bigger and become visible through a normal microscope.

Fungal diseases, above all *Candida albicans*, have been considered difficult to cure. Experiences with grapefruit seed extract can now give hope to many people afflicted with this problem. Doctors and clinics report high success rates with this treatment. The physician Dr. Leo Galland from New York, who has treated many people suffering from chronic *Candida*, only recorded 2 failures among 297 cases. He considers the extract to be "a great breakthrough for patients with chronic fungal and parasitic infections." As an additional bonus, grapefruit seed extract can detoxify the system simultaneously from other fungi and bacteria that often accompany *Candida*, thanks to its broad spectrum of efficacy.

To completely cure *Candida*, grapefruit seed extract should always be employed within the framework of a comprehensive program under competent direction. Without a change of diet, de-toxification of the intestines, reconstruction of healthy intestinal flora, additional strengthening of the immune defenses, and similar measures, the fungi can all too easily overgrow again.

The gradual increase of dosage is particularly important in treating *Candida* since strong toxins are released when the fungi die (Herxheimer's reaction).

Up to now, we have had no practical experience with the use of grapefruit seed extract for *mold*-fungi infections. We therefore can't give any reliable information on dosages. However, laboratory tests have shown great efficacy for the various types of mold fungi. A group of scientists tested grapefruit seed extract on 93 fungal strains and compared it with 18 highly effective customary antimycotics (remedies against fungal infections). The extract proved to be just as effective as the various other agents.

For some years now, grapefruit seed extract has been used against molds on plants and foods. To prevent unintentional ingestion of mold fungi, we recommend that you disinfect fruit, vegetables, and salads in a grapefruit seed extract-water solution for 10 minutes. Mold infestation on damp walls can be stopped with a concentrated solution. (See the chapter "Further Possibilities for Using Grapefruit Seed Extract.")

Dosage guidelines for Candida albicans and other yeast fungi:
1st week: 3 - 9 drops once daily in a glass of water (6 fl. oz.).
2nd week: 3 - 9 drops twice daily in a glass of water (6 fl. oz.).
3rd week: 3 - 9 drops three times daily in a glass of water (6 fl. oz.).

This dose can be changed if the patient doesn't show any Herxheimer's reaction (fatigue, feeling of discomfort, etc.).

The treatment can be continued for 1 - 3 months or longer, according to the intensity and extent of the disease. (Please also refer to the "Instructions for Internal Use.")

Parasitic Diseases

"Make no mistake about it, worms are the most toxic agents in the human body. They are one of the primary underling causes for diseases and are the most basic cause for a compromised immune system." The expert who said this, Dr. Hazel Parcells, is not alone in her opinion. Ann Louise Gittlemann writes: "After more than 18 years of dealing with patients, I am convinced that one of the main causes for the chronically poor health of the people of our age is nothing other than parasites."*

The word "parasite" comes from the Greek language. *Para* means "beside" and *sitos* means "food". A parasite is defined as an organism that lives on or in another organism and feeds at the expense of the host. More than 130 different kinds of parasites use the human being as their host. Their size ranges from the microscopic *protozoa* (single-cell organism) to the meter-long *tapeworm*.

The idea of harboring parasites inside our bodies is repulsive to most people. We tend to deny this possibility and think that the hygienic conditions in our country protect us against parasites. We have learned that parasites only occur in tropical areas or among people who live in unsanitary conditions. However, this is a dangerous misconception since it results not only in a lack of awareness of the risk factors, but also of the symptoms that would indicate an infection with parasites.

Experts consider parasites as the missing diagnosis in the genesis of many chronic health problems. They call it a silent epidemic of which most doctors are not aware. Yet, its recognition will finally solve the mystery of many chronic diseases.

In 1976, the Center for Disease Control (CDC) in America conducted the first and so far only nation-wide survey on the infestation with parasites in the entire population. It revealed that one in every six people selected at random was harboring one or more types of parasites. Dr. Louis Parish determined that at least 8 out of 10 of his patients had a parasitic infection. On the basis of his experiences, he estimates that 25% of the population of New York City is infested. According to other estimations, half of all Americans will become hosts to parasites at one point in their lives.

---

* A. L. Gittlemann: "Guess What Came to Dinner: Parasites and Your Health"

As far as we know, no comparable studies have been done in Europe so far, yet the conditions that have led to a rapid increase of parasitic infections in the USA are the same on our continent:*

- The increase of international travel. It has transformed our planet into a global village, and parasites have developed "wings" as a result.
- The influx of refugees and immigrants from infested areas.
- The keeping of pets that share our living space and often our beds. Pets are hosts to numerous parasites. Dogs can transmit 65 and cats about 40 contageous diseases to human beings.
- The growing popularity of exotic restaurants with raw or undercooked dishes.
- The use of antibiotics or other medications that suppress the immune function.
- The increasing use of day-care centers for babies and toddlers. When the same hands change many diapers, they become a source of contagion. The infection is then very frequently transmitted to parents from the babies.
- The sexual revolution with its practices of anal and oral intercourse and/or frequently changing partners.

The impact of parasitic action is unexpectedly broad. Most invaders live in the **digestive tract**, closely followed by the **blood and lymphatic systems**. Those who live in the intestines, frequently cause digestive problems like **flatulence, constipation,** or **diarrhea**. Parasites often attach themselves to the mucosal lining of the intestines where they leech nutrients from their human host. It is not only the large *tapeworms* that are capable of producing a condition of **malnutrition** with the result of **fatigue, apathy, depressions, lack of concentration, poor memory,** and much more: many smaller parasites can achieve the same effect. Furthermore, parasites can **irritate, inflame,** and **perforate the intestinal lining**. Perforation increases the permeability of the intestinal walls, and large, undigested molecules can pass into the bloodstream. This results in **food allergies** (see "Allergies").

---

* Please understand that this list is not meant to be xenophobic or a moralizing accusation against certain sexual practices.

Beyond the intestines, parasites can settle in the joints and muscles, form cysts, and create inflammations. The resulting pain is often attributed to arthritis. Parasites can even travel into the brain, and they can form granulomes in the lungs, liver, uterus, or other organs. Their toxic metabolic products can attack the central nervous system. Restlessness, depression, and anxiety are often the result.

If parasites penetrate the skin, they often cause rashes, eczema, swelling, papular lesions, skin ulcers, or itching dermatitis.

Parasites can apparently represent a co-factor in the development of AIDS. Researchers at the University of Virginia School of Medicine draw a connection between an epidemic outbreak of amebiasis 2 years prior to the AIDS outbreak in San Francisco. Amoebas produce a substance that ruptures the immune defense cells that enclose and deactivate the HIV virus. Discharged into the bloodstream, the viruses can reproduce unhindered and develop their deadly potential.

The researcher and author Dr. Hulda Regehr Clark (USA) discovered that various *trematodes (flukes)*, among them *intestinal flukes* and *liver flukes*, can cause cancer and other diseases when solvents are present in the body. Normally only the adult stage of these flukes occurs in humans. In the presence of solvents, they can complete all 6 stages of their life cycle within the human body, thereby leaving the organ that they normally colonize and completing their development in some other organ or area of the body. According to Dr. Clark's research, if they begin their reproduction in those inappropriate locations, cancer can form in these areas as a result. The researcher found "misplaced" intestinal flukes in 100% of the cases of cancer she treated. Alzheimer's disease, diabetes, Hodgkin's disease (lymphogranuloma) and much more can also be attributed to "misplaced" flukes.

Since the described process can only take place in the presence of solvents, the author calls it a new type of parasitism, produced by pollution. Solvents are found not only in varnishes, paints, dry-cleaning agents, and synthetic floors. They can be found just as easily in cosmetic preparations like creams, shampoos, soaps, toothpastes, etc., as well as in processed foods. There are a number of ways how solvents can get into processed foods: Traces of solvents can be left from sterilizing the processing and filling equipment; they might be used in the production process; or flavorings or dyes are added that were extracted with the help of solvents. (Dr. Clark points out that the solvent propyl alcohol, which she found within the body in all cancerous diseases, has been used by human beings for about the past 100 years and is therefore just about as old as cancer itself. However, in earlier times it was used much less than today.)

The presence of any kind of parasites leads to an enormous **weakening of the immune system**. Various parasites, such as the widespread protozoa *Giardia lamblia**, reduce the secretion of immunoglobulin A and thereby depress the smooth functioning of our **immune defense**. At the same time, the presence of parasites continuously activates the immune response. This constant "pulling on both ends" can, over time, exhaust our defense system, which is so essential to life.

In addition to the above-mentioned lack of awareness on the part of most doctors regarding the extent of parasitic infections, infestation is difficult to diagnose. Random stool examination—the standard method used by most doctors—has proved to be insufficient and unreliable. On the basis of false negative results, most doctors rule out parasites as the fundamental cause of a disease. Furthermore, the symptoms of an infestation do not always manifest themselves immediately after infection. In many cases, they only appear after days or months have passed.

If a parasitic infection is diagnosed despite these difficulties and treated with medication, new problems may occur because many of the chemicals used in the treatment produce strong side effects.

Grapefruit seed extract is helpful here as well. Not only is it without side effects in contrast to chemical vermifuges, but also extremely effective. A large number of parasitic infections have been successfully treated with the extract. Its broad range of efficacy can also "get us out of the fix" in case of a false diagnosis. For example, if a gastrointestinal parasitic

---

* Dr. Steven Rochlitz writes in his book "Allergies and Candida" that more than 50% of the water supply in the USA is contaminated with *Giardia lamblia* and, unlike bacteria, these protozoa cannot be destroyed with chlorine. We are not aware of any comparable studies in Europe, but it is probable that the same situation applies here.

infection is thought to be caused by bacteria, it will be cured despite the false diagnosis—and without loading our body with useless medication.

In humans, the extract has been principally used against microscopic parasites. However, experiences with animals have shown a clear effect on larger organisms as well.

Dosage: 3 - 15 drops 2 to 3 times daily in accordance with the "Instructions for Internal Use."

Allergies

Allergies are often called one of the modern "plagues." Even babies and toddlers are afflicted by them, and this disease can cause much suffering.

We say that a person is allergic to something when a stimulus that can be completely neutral for others creates a strong defensive reaction. Harmless substances, like pollen, animal hair, food, as well as medications or chemicals, can trigger a response, even in minor doses.

Today it is assumed that a general overloading of the immune system is the main cause for the development of an allergy. Our immune system behaves similarly to a person who always has to "swallow" and "digest" unpleasant experiences. One day, when the burden becomes too great, he finally "overreacts." Certain stimuli act as a "red rag" and drive him mad at the slightest provocation.

Latest research distinguishes between two types of allergies that are characterized by different antibodies, immunoglobulin E (IgE) and immunoglobulin G (IgG). They are sometimes called **primary** and **secondary allergies.** Primary allergies are characterized by a quick onset of clear symptoms like **rashes, swellings**, or **asthma attacks**, developing within a few minutes and up to two hours after contact with the allergen. Even a minor exposure can trigger an immense, sometimes life-threatening reaction.

For many years, allergy research was occupied with this type of allergy alone. However, 70% of the patients who suffer from allergy-like symptoms demonstrate no such immediate reaction and there are also no IgE antibodies in evidence. Their symptoms, known as **food intolerance** or **latent food allergy** among sympathetic therapists, were dismissed by many doctors as imagination or even neurosis.

Only recently has research recognized that these "orphans" among the allergies have their own antibodies, called IgG. With the help of a special blood test*, these allergies can now be recognized and accurately diagnosed. Without such an aid, a **secondary allergy** is difficult to determine since the reaction is delayed—anywhere from hours to days after indulgence in the respective food.

Two basic conditions are responsible for the development of a **secondary allergy**, whose antigen is always a food: insufficient production of hydrochloric acid in the stomach and a "leaky gut." The lack of stomach acid leads to inadequate pre digestion, and proteins, the most difficult molecules to digest, are not properly broken down. If the intestinal wall proves to have gaps that are too large, the undigested food molecules pass into the bloodstream, where they are seen as foreign and treated accordingly.

The B-lymphocytes of the immune system now begin to detoxify the "food poisons." For this purpose, they produce the above-mentioned IgG antibodies that attach themselves to the molecules so that they can be identified. If all goes well, these food-IgG complexes are eaten up by the white immune cells. If there are too many, however, the body deposits them in joints, muscles, skin, brain, lungs, arteries, or just about anywhere in the body. This leads to **dysfunctions, inflammations, pain, degeneration**, or **water retention** in the affected areas. Furthermore, the immune systems uses up a large portion of its capacity in the battle against these "food poisons" so that it is poorly equipped to fight infections.

The **secondary food allergy** can be responsible for a very wide range of symptoms. More than 50 conditions and 200 symptoms have been reported so far. The symptoms can occur in almost every organ or tissue. Some of the most frequent are **headaches** or **chronic migraines, fatigue, diarrhea, constipation, flatulence, Crohn's disease, colitis, eczema,**

---

* ELISA blood test = "Enzyme Linked Immuno Sorbant Assay." See Appendix under "Supply Sources" for institute addresses.

nettle rash (hives), **asthma**, as well as different kinds of **rheumatism**. In countless cases, these and many other symptoms disappeared or at least improved considerably when the respective food was eliminated from the diet.

People with **primary allergies** against pollen, animal hair, house dust, certain foods, etc. found their reactions greatly reduced as soon as they recovered from their **secondary allergies**. They now required a much stronger exposure to trigger an attack.

Insufficient production of hydrochloric acid can be caused by hurried meals, stress and anxiety, certain medications, old age, and alcohol abuse. Further causes are **inflammations in the gastrointestinal tract** due to *parasites, Candida albicans,* or other *micro-organisms*.

If an **inflammation** exists in the intestines, a reflex switches off the production of hydrochloric acid in the stomach. Mother Nature urges us to fast, but we usually don't listen. Due to the lack of stomach acid, pre-digestion is insufficient and over-sized molecules pass into the intestines. If they meet with a "leaky gut," the described process begins.

The most frequent causes of a "leaky gut" are antibiotics and pain-killers, alcohol, an unbalanced diet, bottle-feeding and solid foods before the 6th month of life, as well as **infections** through *parasites, Helicobacter pylori* and *Candida albicans*. If, for example, the *Candida* yeast fungus "overgrows," it develops long threads that grow like roots through the intestinal wall and perforate it. The bites of parasites can have a similar effect.

As already mentioned, symptoms can be markedly reduced or disappear if we remove the respective foods from our diet. The memory of B-lymphocytes, which trigger production of IgG, only lasts for 2 - 3 months. If we stop eating the food for 3 months, we can then usually take it again without any allergic reaction.

However, we will develop a new onset of food intolerances if we do not eliminate the fundamental conditions that triggered our food allergy in the first place.

Grapefruit seed extract can help us to free the afflicted stomach and intestinal walls of parasites, bacteria, and fungi. The elimination of the toxic strain that accompanies **food allergies** can unburden the immune system to such an extent that even

primary allergies nearly or completely disappear. Furthermore, a relieved immune system can much more effectively master its other tasks.

Dosage: See the respective chapters on infection by bacteria, fungi, or parasites.

Prevention is Better than Cure

After we have seen how easily pathogens—whether they are bacteria, viruses, fungi, or parasites—get into our body and how much havoc they can wreak, the question may arise: "Wouldn't it be smart to take a few drops of grapefruit seed extract every day as a preventative against the uninvited guests? Since it's non-toxic, it can't do any harm but will be very beneficial."

Everyone has to answer this question individually, but we want to provide some information to help you make this decision.

To date there are no known side effects, even when the extract is used for a long time. It was reported that Dr. Harich, the discoverer of grapefruit seed extract, has taken 2 drops every morning for the past 13 years as a preventative. At the age of 70, he is still jetting around the world to organize his international operations.

The organic farmer Knud Dencker-Jensen, who distributes grapefruit seed extract in Denmark to both horticultural and livestock farms, told us about a farmer's wife who has taken a teaspoon of the extract every day for the past year and has never felt so healthy in her life. Its astonishing effect on her animals had inspired her to this "therapy," and it wasn't too long before other women in her neighborhood followed her example. We don't want to recommend such a high dose, but this example demonstrates the harmlessness of the extract, even in high doses over extended periods of time.

Various doctors prescribe continuous administration for one year or longer in special cases, such as preventative measures for patients with recurring vaginitis. The physician Dr. Leo Galland of New York reports that even when ingested for twelve months, the extract showed no side effects. Furthermore, none of his patients developed immune resistance. The latter is a problem that can occur when antibiotics are frequently ingested. Grapefruit seed extract appears to keep its effect, even when used for a long period of time.

We think that prevention is not necessary where the immune system is intact. However, if our immune system is weakened or chronic illnesses have taken hold, a few drops of grapefruit seed extract every day can be very helpful. Beside its curative effect, it can protect us from the additional stress placed on our immune system by acute infections.

All the same, we would like to discourage you from giving babies and toddlers the extract on a continuous basis as a preventative. At birth, our immune system has not yet fully developed and must practice to acquire its ability to protect us from disease. If we take the possibility of "practicing" away from a child at an early age, by the too hasty and repeated administration of antibiotics, fever-reducing agents, and vaccinations, the immune system can only develop inadequately. For the same reason, taking grapefruit seed extract on a continuous basis wouldn't be appropriate either. Yet, the extract can represent a wonderful, harmless alternative to antibiotics or other medications in the case of illness. The child's sensitive intestinal flora remains intact and no side effects occur when used properly.

However, taking the extract as a preventative measure is recommended on trips to distant countries. See the chapter "The Smallest Portable Medicine chest in the World" on this topic. Also when a wave of influenza is advancing or a "tummy bug" goes around, prevention with grapefruit seed extract can effectively protect us from contagion.

The Smallest Portable Medicine Chest in the World

An ounce of prevention is worth a pound of cure

- PROVERB -

How many of us have already experienced this: the long-awaited vacation in a foreign country finally begins, but instead of enjoying the sun and the beautiful landscape, we are plagued by diarrhea. If your travels take you to Asia, Africa, or South America, you may have to boil your drinking water or disinfect it with chlorine every day in order not to get anything worse than simple diarrhea. Uncooked food is also taboo or must be chlorinated since some uninvited guests may all too easily slip into our body together with the fresh tomatoes. But even these precautions are no guarantee if we inadvertently moisten our toothbrush with tap water.

If, after such a journey, someone told you: "On your next trip you can forget all about it, drink the water, eat what you like, and enjoy your vacation," you may only reply with a tired smile. Yet, grapefruit seed extract has proved to be a wonderful, simple alternative. Various doctors recommend drinking 3 to 5 drops of the extract in a glass of water every day as a preventative—and enjoy the foreign culinary pleasures without complaints.

Dr. C. W. Lynn of Orlando, Florida, had an interesting experience in this respect. He traveled with a group of 38 patients to Mexico and South America. Half of the group took 3 drops of grapefruit seed extract every day. None of them became ill, while the entire other half of the group came down with diarrhea.

If you travel into countries where hygienic conditions are very poor and life-threatening infections are still a daily occurrence, we advise that you disinfect your drinking water and wash or soak fruits and salads, as well as your eating utensils, in disinfected water for several minutes. For this purpose, grapefruit seed extract is a healthy substitute for chlorine, which is known to have side effects. A dilution of about 200 ppm which corresponds to 18 drops in one liter (35 fl. oz.) of water is usually sufficient for disinfection. Or you can simply put a few drops into a glass of drinking water. Before drinking, mix the extract well and give it a few minutes to take effect. The slightly bitter taste of the grapefruit seed extract is usually willingly accepted.

If drinks are served with ice-cubes, you should remember that these can often be germ-transmitters, as studies in many countries have shown. A few drops of grapefruit seed extract will guarantee protection from infection. Don't forget to add a few drops of extract to the water you use for brushing your teeth. Your teeth and gums will be grateful as well.

The water-purifying effect of grapefruit seed extract can also be a great help for adventurers who want to explore areas far away from civilization where water doesn't flow from the tap. Even in untouched regions, the water from streams and lakes isn't necessarily "safe." A filter usually means an unpleasant burden in the baggage and doesn't always keep the promise that it makes. Here also a few drops of grapefruit seed extract are a welcome alternative. The exact dosage has already been mentioned above. If the water contains many particles of dirt, it should be filtered beforehand through a fine cloth.

If we have contracted an illness while travelling, the extract serves as an effective aid. Not only will the flu that has just now got hold of us be cured more quickly, but also the many unaccustomed bacteria that we come into contact with while travelling won't be able to make themselves at home within our body. In case of an illness, it is recommended that you take 3 - 15 drops 2 to 3 times daily in a glass of water until the symptoms have disappeared. (For further information see "Instructions for Internal Use.")

Furthermore, grapefruit seed extract may come in handy against many other complaints that we may catch during our travels. Thanks to its antiseptic, germ-killing, and fungicidal effect it always presents itself as an interesting universal remedy for not just gastrointestinal upsets, parasitic infestation, or sore throat, but also for bothersome athlete's foot, insect stings, scrapes, cuts, or bite wounds. As "coincidence" would have it, one of our American publishers called us one evening and mentioned among other things his upcoming lecturing trip through a number of countries. We wished him all the best and that he may return home in good health. "Of course," he said with conviction, "for some time, I've been using a certain grapefruit seed extract on all my trips—I don't think you've heard about it yet. I've had no health problems on my trips since." He had no idea that we were just writing a book about this wonderful extract.

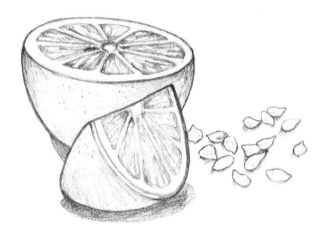

Reports on Experiences

Woman from Bantry: "I have suffered from mouth ulcers for some years now. The various remedies only had a temporary effect or none at all. A friend recommended grapefruit seed extract to me, and I rinsed my mouth with it several times a day. There was a distinct improvement after 24 hours, and after 48 hours my complaint had disappeared. What a relief after such a long time. I could hardly believe it. Now I rinse my mouth with grapefruit seed extract regularly after brushing my teeth, and the mouth ulcer hasn't returned."

Woman from Castletown: "I often had a problem with bladder infections and when it got very bad two months ago, I finally took the strong antibiotic that my doctor had prescribed once again. I felt very wretched afterwards. A short time later, the same bladder complaint came back and I was close to despair since there was blood in the urine again and the pain became unbearable—what could help now? When you brought me the bottle of grapefruit seed extract, I honestly didn't have much hope, but then out of sheer desperation I took the drops like you told me to. To my surprise, the blood in the urine and the strong pain when urinating disappeared within a few hours. However, I still had slight symptoms for about a week. Since I saw no other way, I decided to go back to the doctor to get some more antibiotics. I called and made an appointment for the next day. However, to my great surprise I was completely without symptoms the next morning, so I cancelled the appointment for the time being. To this day (3 weeks later), the bladder inflammation hasn't returned. It finally appears to be cured—I would like to thank you very much for the grapefruit remedy."

(*Note by the authors:* Because of the previous use of antibiotics, her body probably needed longer to recover. Even after 3 months, the young woman's symptoms haven't returned.)

Young man from Bantry: "I would like to tell you about an amazing experience with grapefruit seed extract. Since childhood I have had severe asthma attacks that even increased over the years. I finally had to go straight to hospital with every attack and would usually stay there for a week. I tried the grapefruit seed extract without great expectations. When there were signs of a new attack, they suddenly subsided, and I could stay at home. I continue to take the extract regularly and am curious to see how things will go. Up to now, I have been spared any new attacks."

Alan C. from Cork: "After years of futile attempts with diets and other remedies, grapefruit seed extract cured me of Candida albicans. I have never felt so fresh and well all around. My constant urge for sweets has also disappeared. My wife, who also suffered from Candida, had a similar wonderful experience. I am really grateful that something like this exists."

Young woman from Glengarriff: "Since my pregnancy 8 years ago, I've had a persistent fungal infection in the vagina. I tried remedies from the pharmacy, alternative remedies like aloe vera and tea tree oil, but the success never lasted long. When I heard of grapefruit seed extract, I rinsed my vagina with a solution of water and grapefruit seed extract. I also inserted a tampon that I had soaked in the solution and left it overnight. After a few days, the itching stopped, but I continued the treatment for another 10 days in order to be sure. At the same time, I took the remedy orally. To my surprise, my digestive complaints improved. I can finally enjoy sex again and the bothersome itch hasn't returned."

Thomas B. from Frankfurt/M.: "The eczema on my scalp has disappeared—at last after six years. I only used the grapefruit seed extract twice and I have no problems anymore."

Farmer from Skibbereen: "One day, a round, itching, red spot, which we call ringworm, (a fungal infection caused by a microspore from the genus Fungi Imperfecti), developed on the skin of my leg. The cows often have this fungus, and on a farm it's easy to get infected. I had always used something from the pharmacy, but this time a friend gave me a little bottle of grapefruit seed extract. So I rubbed some on my leg, twice a day of course, like I always did with the stuff from the pharmacy. I know how stubborn these things are, but this time it disappeared more quickly than any other time. It's really great that something from nature helps so well."

Nurse from Cork: "I must say that grapefruit seed extract has changed my life. For many years, I had an ulcer on my leg. It was constantly open, and I had to always wear a bandage as protection against infection and go regularly to the hospital for treatment. The pain often kept me awake at night, so I had to take pain-killers all the time. When they finally told me at the hospital that my leg might have to be amputated, I was really in despair. At that time I was taking care of an old lady, and her son knew about herbs. In my desperation I poured out my troubles to him. He mixed a tincture for me and said I should soak the bandage for my leg with it every day. The tincture contained some herbs, but my leg hardly improved. He tried out different things and one day he told me that he had a new remedy, grapefruit seed extract, that he wanted to add to the other things. The pain had already gotten less through aloe vera, but the new remedy worked real wonders. Although I still have the ulcer today, the infection has healed for the first time in 9 years. I sleep very well without pills once again. I have no pain anymore and no longer need to go to the hospital for treatment. I was able to keep my leg. What a blessing. I thank God for this miracle."

Olivia K. from Regensburg: "One of my toes had hurt for several days and when I finally checked it, the area around the nail was swollen and reddened. It looked like a panaritium. Since I had already used grapefruit seed extract for a Candida albicans infection in my intestines and vagina with great success, I also tried it here and dabbed the spot about 4 times with the extract. I then forgot about my toe since it didn't cause any more trouble. When I remembered it after a few days and checked it again, the redness and swelling had disappeared. What a great remedy! I recommend it to all my friends."

John S. from Killarney: "For more than ten years I had athlete's foot between several toes. No matter what ointments, sprays, and powders I tried, this fungus never totally disappeared. During the last few months, it even started to spread further. The advice of trying a grapefruit seed solution was just one of many in recent years. Yet, to my own surprise, for the first time it seems that my athlete's foot has finally disappeared. My mother has also washed my socks with grapefruit seed extract for the last few weeks, to prevent reinfection.

Dorit K. from Munich: "For many years, I can hardly remember how long, I had bleeding gums that were receding more and more from my crowned front teeth. Nothing helped. Finally, the roots of the teeth were showing and tooth decay started. It looked horrible. I no longer dared to laugh out loud and tried to hide the ugly rims above my teeth as well as possible. In long sessions at the dentist I received new crowns that covered the roots of the teeth and the gums were cut and sewed. Some weeks after this awful procedure, my gums began to bleed again and wouldn't stop. Had the whole thing started all over again? I was very lucky to become acquainted with grapefruit seed extract shortly afterwards. A girlfriend from Ireland had sent it to me. Every day I put a few drops on my toothbrush and a few drops into the water I use for rinsing after brushing my teeth. The bleeding stopped almost immediately and hasn't returned once. I now have the feeling that I can laugh out loud until the end of my life."

A young boy from our neighborhood: Several weeks ago, a neighbor came to us for help on a Sunday. Her seven-year-old son had a bad infection behind his ear. The mother said, "At first it was probably just a skin fungus behind the ear that itched terribly. Because of the scratching, it turned into a festering, oozing infection about as large as the palm of my hand." The ear was so stuck to the scalp that it was a painful and dramatic moment as we tried to separate scalp, hair, and ear from each other. Normally we would have taken the boy to a clinic, but since we live far out in the Irish countryside and there was no means of transportation available except a motorcycle, we decided to treat him ourselves. We covered the entire wound with grapefruit seed extract powder in order to dry out the oozing infection and prevent the ear from sticking to the scalp again. The next day his mother called and said, "Thank God, the whole wound is dry and crusted today. It appears to be healing." – Powder was put on it for the following four days. Then came another call, "It's now completely healed, it's like a miracle, not even a scar is left behind—how can I thank you?"

Paul M. from Baltimore: "As a professional diver, I've had slight athlete's foot for many years, but now this fungus had spread to above my knees so that my girlfriend wanted to leave me. All the stuff from the pharmacy was just rubbish, nothing really helped. Then I tried grapefruit seed extract, although I didn't dilute it as recommended but simply rubbed it on. It worked wonders. Could I have a few more bottles for my colleagues?"

(Although we like to pass on a bottle of grapefruit seed extract occasionally, it comes from our private supply—and since we are not doctors, we can only give advice to personal friends and acquaintances.)

Laura O. from Clear Island: "Last year an intestinal disease was rampant in our area a number of times and I was always among the afflicted. But ever since I started taking a few drops of grapefruit seed extract at the slightest sign of an intestinal infection, I never had any trouble again."

Sandy F. from Cork: "What is a singer without a voice? Should I take antibiotics again?" Sandy asked us before her concert, seeking help. She gargled several times with some grapefruit seed extract—that we luckily had in our pocket— and the problem was soon forgotten. "It is wonderful, I feel great, yes, I feel good now—thank you!"

Further Possibilities for Using Grapefruit Seed Extract

In Personal Hygiene

Almost every personal hygiene product can complete its task even more effectively with a small addition of grapefruit seed extract. The extract provides additional freshness and cleanliness in the care of teeth, skin, and hair and can protect us from unpleasant body odors. To eliminate or prevent these odors, chemical agents are often used, which can irritate the skin and also enter the body by penetrating the skin through the pores. Above all, the extract can prevent certain diseases.

Adding grapefruit seed extract to liquid soap or shower gel thoroughly disinfects the skin and protects it against skin and nail fungi. Used in the genital area, the antiseptic effect of the extract can prevent infections and undesirable odors without irritating the sensitive mucous membranes. In shampoo, it helps against dandruff, itchy scalp, and eczema. We recommend the addition of 10 - 20 drops to 100 ml (3.5 fl. oz.) of the respective personal hygiene product. Two drops of the extract on a moist toothbrush keep teeth and gums healthy. The extract can also be used as an effective antiseptic mouthwash that keeps the breath fresh for a long time and is a beneficial additive to your "water pik."

Many people report that the sweaty condition of their feet disappeared in a very short time, often after just one application of the extract. For this purpose, the extract can be sprayed, rubbed in, or added to the foot bath. (For all these applications, also see the chapter "Grapefruit Seed Extract for External Use").

In order to prevent underarm odor caused by bacteria in the armpits, you can create your own deodorant spray in a simple way. Pour a cup of water with 15 - 20 drops of grapefruit seed extract into an empty spray bottle. Shake well and spray under the arms. This eliminates the annoying odor in a comfortable way.

If you don't want to enrich your personal hygiene products with grapefruit seed extract yourself, you can now buy an entire range of ready-made products. In addition to a large number of preparations for health and general hygiene, more and more cosmetic articles and personal hygiene products are being produced containing this effective extract. Soaps, shower and body gels, shampoos, toothpastes, skin creams and sprays, as well as bath and deodorant products, containing grapefruit seed extract are now all available.

A surge of interest in grapefruit seed extract has been observed in the USA. Health food stores and some of the larger organic trade chains have switched over to grapefruit seed extract products. Observers of economic trends have already evaluated the new extract as a biological marketing sensation.

While we were working on this book, every few weeks news flowed in about a further personal hygiene product based on grapefruit seed extract. This reflects a change in people's awareness, which motivates manufacturers to produce articles that not only provide optimal care, but are beneficial for our health and safe for the environment.

In Cosmetics

Pore-deep cleansing is a precondition for healthy, glowing skin. Part of this means freeing the skin from undesirable bacteria that can produce pimples, pustules, or inflammations. An increasing number of cosmeticians and beauty therapists use grapefruit seed extract for this purpose with great success.

The antiseptic effect of the extract can also be very helpful for acne. Customary acne agents often contain substances that attack the skin. Even if pimples sprout merrily during puberty, grapefruit seed extract can create welcome relief. After the removal of blackheads and other skin impurities, as well as the plucking or shaving of unwanted hairs, the extract provides excellent disinfection.

For a thorough cleansing of your face, spread a few drops of grapefruit seed extract on your wet hands and massage into the moistened skin (also see the chapter "Grapefruit Seed Extract for External Use" on this topic). *Avoid contact with the eyes.* In case of emergency, rinse the eyes with lots of water.

There is yet another area of use for grapefruit seed extract in cosmetics. We would like to relate a little incident in this regard.

"For a long time now I've had this eczema on my face and I can't get rid of it. It keeps coming back. Do you know anything that could help?" Our friend Gaby, who called us from Germany, sounded quite desperate. We had just discovered grapefruit seed extract for ourselves and advised her to try it. However, with further questioning we discovered that she was using a home-made natural cosmetic—with wonderful ingredients and, in order to avoid undesirable chemicals, without any preservatives. A big jar had been mixed for her which lasted a long time. "This is already two years old," she now determined with slight alarm. Right after our conversation, she tossed the jar into the garbage and had a new mixture made—this time with grapefruit seed extract as a preservative... and surprise, the eczema disappeared after a short time.

Many people create their own cosmetic articles today. The opinion that artificial products from the chemical factory don't belong on the skin has become increasingly widespread. Television shows, courses, books, and magazine articles inform the public on the topic of "making natural cosmetics yourself," and in almost every city there is a store offering the necessary basic substances. At the same time, the professional field of biological cosmetics is booming like never before. More and more large manufacturers are joining the trend, even those who used to shake their heads about it.

Natural cosmetics often have a big disadvantage that is frequently given too little consideration. The lack of preservatives, both in commercial cosmetics and self-mixed preparations, creates the ideal breeding ground for bacteria and fungi. The micro-organisms can very easily get into the product by way of the fingers. Even if a cosmetic preparation contains exquisite substances, it can turn into an unhealthy product through the inadvertent introduction of undesirable micro-organisms.

As long as a preservative doesn't guarantee sterility, favorable survival conditions for a broad spectrum of germs dominate in most cosmetics: a good breeding ground, sufficient moisture, relative darkness, and enough time to develop.

For preservation purposes, grapefruit seed extract is usually added in a concentration between 0.2% and 1%. It can easily be worked into the aqueous phase and can also be processed with organic solvents, butylene alcohol, and alcohol. The extract should always be mixed well into the preparation. In terms of what ingredients to use, there are no limits to your imagination. You can continue to use all of the active substances previously employed.

After the discovery of grapefruit seed extract and the first reports on its effectiveness, manufacturers of natural cosmetics quickly realized what was being offered to them: an extract that, due to its inhibitory effect on a broad spectrum of bacteria, fungi, and viruses, was not only suitable for preservation, but also possessed wonderful skin care properties. A positive side effect of using cosmetics preserved with grapefruit seed extract was observed: unwanted eczema, skin fungi, herpes, rashes, lip blisters, and other skin problems simply disappeared. This means that grapefruit seed extract not only keeps cosmetics healthy, but also helps those who use them to achieve better health.

In Baby Care

The special qualities of grapefruit seed extract make it suitable for the delicate skin of a baby's bottom as well as the sensitive internal organs of our youngest residents on Earth. There are many ways that this extract can be used for baby care.

Many babies suffer from yeast fungal infections (saccharomycosis) in the mouth and diaper area, commonly known as thrush or diaper rash. Thrush can be seen as a whitish coating in the mouth. When our son suffered from it as a baby, the doctor prescribed a remedy, which we later heard to be a suspected carcinogen. We didn't know about grapefruit seed extract at that time. Without doubt, it would have been the remedy of our choice.

In the case of a thrush infection, a harmless alternative is particularly desirable since the remedy is put directly into the mouth. For treatment, mix half a capsule of the powder, which is less bitter than the drops, into a cup of water. Then paint the mouth—as well as possible—with the solution. Somewhat older children can also gargle with the mixture. The addition of fruit juice can largely neutralize the bitter taste.

To disinfect baby-bottle nipples and pacifiers, add 20 drops of grapefruit seed extract to 1 liter (35 fl. oz.) of water and leave them in the solution for 20 minutes. This method prevents reinfection, as well as new infections with other germs. Rinse well afterwards. Bitter isn't exactly the favorite flavor of babies.

Today most babies are wrapped in plastic diapers that make care much easier, but permit no air to reach their bottoms. Moisture, darkness, and warmth let the germs grow, particularly the yeast fungus *Candida albicans*, which produces the so-called diaper rash. Even the greatest absorbent power of disposable diapers apparently isn't sufficient to completely prevent its spread. The good old cloth diapers have proved to be the best solution here.

We can get even the most stubborn diaper rash under control with grapefruit seed extract, although a bit of patience is sometimes required. Put about 10 drops in an egg-cup of oil and gently rub it into the skin. It is advisable to switch to cloth diapers until the problem has healed. The baby's bottom should also get as much fresh air as possible.

If you use washable cloth diapers add 20 drops of grapefruit seed extract to the last rinse. Hot water temperatures do not always kill the fungi completely.

If you don't want to part with the practical plastic diapers you can dust the inside of them with a thin layer of grapefruit seed extract powder. We haven't tried this out, but we assume that diaper rash can be prevented in this way.

Furthermore, objects that babies frequently put in their mouths can be disinfected with a solution of 20 drops of grapefruit seed extract in 1 liter (35 fl. oz.) of water. Leave them in the solution for 10 minutes and then let them dry in the air. However, we should also remember that exposure to germs is natural and will stimulate the baby's immune system. We wish you and your babies much happiness and inner contentment in a healthy skin!

In Nursing Care

All patients require special attention and Tender Loving Care together with general medical care and support. In addition to other measures, the weakened organism should be protected from undesirable germs. In the case of a contagious disease, protecting the care-giver from infection is also necessary.

We've already reported on the successful use of grapefruit seed extract in hospitals as a disinfectant, which is also relevant when providing nursing-care at home. To disinfect the patient's room, add grapefruit seed extract to the various cleaning agents. The patient's bed linen, clothing, and towels can be washed with the addition of 20 drops of extract to the last rinse. Objects that the patient touches can also be disinfected with the help of grapefruit seed extract. For this purpose, add 30 to 40 drops of extract to 1 liter (35 fl. oz.) of water and place the objects in it for several minutes. They can also be washed with the solution. If we want to improve the air in the patient's room, we can put the same solution in a spray bottle and atomize it. The extract can be used as an effective germ-inhibitor in both air-humidifiers and artificial ventilating systems.

Care-givers are advised to disinfect their hands with the extract before and after contact with the patient. Nurses and doctors sometimes suffer from eczema on their hands, caused by the caustic chemical disinfectants. The use of grapefruit seed extract for disinfecting the hands not only prevents this occurrence, but also helps heal existing eczema. For disinfection purposes, put a few drops of the extract directly on the moist hands and rub it in.

Not only is grapefruit seed extract harmless for this purpose as well, but also extremely effective. In a previous chapter we mentioned the study by Dr. J. A. Botine determining that the extract has a 100% disinfectant effect in comparison to the 98% of the usual agent and the 72% efficacy of alcohol. What has been a swab with alcohol before an injection or the prick of an acupuncture needle, could soon be the swab with grapefruit seed extract. The chemical pre-operative and post-operative skin disinfection currently used could also be advantageously replaced with the extract. In addition, plasters or bandage materials could be pre-treated by spraying them with grapefruit seed extract.

Doctors, naturopaths, midwives, nurses, chiropodists, and others who are involved with the treatment and care of patients may find many other uses for grapefruit seed extract. The extract can be used wherever an antibacterial, antiseptic, or fungicidal effect is required.

As a Household Aid

Throughout the entire world, the majority of jobs are found in the household. Seen in global terms, no other area of work has as many part-time and full-time workers. Above all, these workers are responsible for cleanliness and food—for themselves as well as the people entrusted to them. A great portion of our physical well-being comes from this source.

Many cleaning agents and detergents contain disinfecting chemicals. This fact reflects our need to keep our domestic environment not only looking clean, but also free of germs. Whenever small children or pets share our living space with us, this is particularly important. Bacteria, viruses, fungi, and parasites can be carried into our home by shoes and clothing, pets, foods, and visitors, and enter our bodies through physical contact or consumption.

If they meet with an intact immune system, they usually don't cause any damage. However, most people today are no longer adequately armed against the many invaders. Stress, improper diets, antibiotics, and other things have weakened our immune system. Therefore, prevention is advisable. Yet, the chemicals used for disinfection are not only strong or even caustic, but frequently also very toxic. Fortunately, nature has given us a helper in this situation that is powerful, organic, and safe for health: the extract from the seed of the grapefruit. Since it is neither toxic nor caustic, it can also be used in those areas where disinfection by chemicals could lead to health damage or might attack materials.

Grapefruit seed extract can therefore be added to almost every cleaning or disinfection process: when washing dishes by hand and in the dishwasher, for surface cleaning of furniture and floors, in the kitchen, bathroom, or toilet, for cleaning carpets and washing laundry. A broad spectrum of bacteria, viruses, fungi, and microscopic parasites can be eliminated by adding 20 - 30 drops of liquid grapefruit seed extract to a basin of water. We add about 50 drops of the extract to a bucket of floor-cleaning water or about 15 drops to a spray bottle, so that it can also be sprayed. About 20 drops can be added to the last rinse in the washer, as well as to the dishwasher. Chopping and cutting boards can also be effectively sterilized with grapefruit seed extract. This is particularly important when raw meat, one of the most frequent sources of parasitic infections, is prepared on them. Allow the extract to take effect for several minutes, then rinse off.

Not only raw meat, poultry, fish, and shellfish are transmitters of germs, but also salads, vegetables, and fruits can pass on a great number of bacteria, mold, or parasites. If we add 20 drops of grapefruit seed extract to one liter (35 fl. oz.) of water and place the foods into this solution for a few minutes, not only will the undesired germs and parasites be killed, but the shelf life of the foods will be increased at the same time. The formation of rot and the very toxic mold fungi is delayed for quite a while.

We love to eat papayas, which we can only order by the crate from the supermarket in the nearest town. This means we have to keep them for a long time. These delicious fruits seem to mold more quickly than any other fruit. Since we started to rub some drops of full-strength extract on our papayas, not even the last papaya in the crate has gone moldy. You can also try preserving home-made jam with grapefruit seed extract.

In addition to cleaning applications and food, there are some further areas in which the extract can be usefully employed. We can, for example, prevent microbic contamination or the growth of algae in **air-humidifiers** and **air dehumidifiers, air-conditioning systems**, or **indoor fountains**. A few drops of grapefruit seed extract in the watering can for house plants eliminates any mold on their soil. Adding it to your **hydroponic system** will prevent the formation of molds there as well.

Thanks to its bacteria-inhibiting and fungicidal quality, grapefruit seed extract is an interesting way to keep cut flowers fresh. For this purpose, put one-half to one capsule of the grapefruit seed extract powder into the flower-water (according to the size of the vase) and mix well. The liquid extract is not suitable for this purpose since it is combined with glycerine, which can close off the fine supply channels in the stem of the flower. Please cut off the ends of the flower stems before putting them in the vase. The commercially available preparations for this purpose contain sugar as a nutrient in addition to germ-inhibitors and algae-inhibitors. If we also add a small portion of sugar to our mixture, we can extend our enjoyment of the flowers in a simple way.

In the Catering Trade and Food Industry

Have you ever sat in a bar or restaurant and observed how many beerglasses travel through the same sink in order to be immediately filled with beer again? You might have noticed a beer-drinking, coughing neighbor to your right and sneezing neighbor to your left and secretly wished that the water in the sink might contain an effective disinfectant.

Glasses, silverware, and dishes that are used by many different people, as they are in the catering trade, are always a potential source for the spreading of germs. Because of their unhealthy effects, chemicals can't be used for disinfection. So the use of grapefruit seed extract would be particularly worthwhile in this case.

Studies have shown time and again that beer pipes—from the barrel to the tap—are a breeding-ground for countless germ cultures. A routine cleaning with the addition of grapefruit seed extract could also be recommended here.

Further areas of use for grapefruit seed extract in the catering trade and the hotel business correspond to those in the private household. We would like to ask our readers to see the chapter "As a Household Aid" for further suggestions.

There are also many interesting possible uses for grapefruit seed extract in the food and beverage industries. How many new substances and sophisticated, ingenious processes are constantly being developed in order to increase the shelf life of products? From the producers point of view this is quite understandable since their products can only be marketed if they appear to be fresh and unspoiled. Consumers, on the other hand, need healthy and high-quality foods whose life-enhancing qualities have not been destroyed. The producers' attitude ignores this requirement. More and more non-food ingredients are added to preserve and visually enhance the food. Others are added to make it more convenient to prepare at home. By doing this, the vital substances contained in the food can be destroyed.

These measures are concealed from the customer's eye to a great degree. Even if he makes the effort to decipher the list of additives, he will often only find those additives that must be listed according to law. Furthermore, many additives only have to be listed if a certain amount is exceeded. Some manufacturers circumvent this requirement, particularly regarding questionable substances, by staying just below this threshold. Many people have become accustomed to industrially processed foods without any awareness of how alien this type of diet is to a natural life. Others, however, have a deep sense of uneasiness when faced with the increasing amount of industrially processed foods.

Food should always be eaten in its natural form, and as fresh as possible. Nevertheless, we must admit that some form of preservation is required at times. Relatively few foods are available to us in a fresh form during both the summer and the winter. And if we want to enjoy the delicious taste of oranges from South America, kiwis from New Zealand, bananas from Africa, or pineapples from the Caribbean, then we must ask ourselves how the wide distances should be bridged without the fruits spoiling.

In South America, grapefruit seed extract is already used to a large extent for the preservation of fruit, vegetables, nuts, fish, and meat. A spray procedure is usually employed for this purpose. In an experiment, it was possible to extend the shelf life of fruits and vegetables three to four times with the help of grapefruit seed extract. Mold and rot can be prevented in an extremely effective manner, and the food survives a longer transportation time without damage. Consumers of foods treated with the extract are also protected from the transmission of disease-causing germs that are increasingly spreading throughout the world by the transportation of fruit and other foods.

Some of the preservative substances in the food-processing industry could be replaced by grapefruit seed extract. This would reduce the strain on our bodies caused by foreign substances. The powder would be better suited for this purpose since it is less bitter and should hardly impair the taste. The amounts that may get into our bodies as a result should do more to promote good health than to harm it. Remember that we would have to ingest about 3 liters (at a concentration of 33% active substances and 80 kilograms of body weight) before we would poison ourselves.

We can well imagine that future advertising will read "Preserved only with Grapefruit Seed Extract" or that there will even be a "Grapefruit Seed Bio-Seal" in order to show customers that a product contains no artificial preservatives. However, there is still much research work to be done before this can happen.

Cleanliness is also a high priority in the food industry. Processing machines and filling equipment have to adhere to the required hygienic standards. Residues from disinfectants used for this purpose can get into processed or filled foods and cause damage to our health.

The researcher and author Dr. Hulda Regehr Clark discovered that in all the cases of cancer she treated, the solvent isopropyl alcohol was evident in the patients' bodies. In her opinion, this agent participates substantially in the development of cancer and a range of other diseases. Other solvents are said to play a similar role in the development of further diseases. (See the chapter "Grapefruit Seed Extract for Inner Use.") We presume that these agents are used for the disinfection of processing and filling facilities. From there, they get into beverages and foods and continue on into the human body.

Our organism is already over-burdened by the many foreign substances added to our food. This load could be significantly reduced through the use of a biological disinfectant and cleaning agent. We hope that the responsible parties will take up this idea and put it into practice for the benefit of many people.

In the Sauna, Whirlpool, and Swimming Pool

The **sauna**, especially the public sauna, is a rich breeding ground for fungi because of its construction, the climatic conditions (wood, heat, moisture, relative darkness), and many different users. This applies primarily to the lower area of the sauna where temperatures aren't too hot. On the upper benches, the air temperature ranging from 140 to 203 degrees F. assures that most of these cultures are killed. Another problem is that the interior of the sauna with its many individual parts is very difficult to clean or disinfect.

The use of chemical cleaning or hygienic agents has several disadvantages. On one hand, residues can irritate the skin and get into the body through the pores. On the other hand, the cleaning agent may evaporate when the sauna is heated, giving off toxic vapors, which can get into the lungs when inhaled. The use of grapefruit seed extract with its fungicidal and antibacterial effect offers an interesting and welcome alternative.

The simplest approach is to spray diluted grapefruit seed extract using a spray bottle, but surfaces can just as effectively be wiped off with a solution. About 20 drops of the 60% basic extract in a liter (35 fl. oz.) of water is enough to achieve a powerful effect and eliminate almost all known bacteria, germs, and fungi. It is best to clean the sauna when it is unheated. The floor can be sprayed or wiped with the same solution.

By using grapefruit seed extract in place of chemical disinfectants, possible skin irritations can be avoided. Furthermore, test studies in the USA have shown that grapefruit seed extract, if inhaled as a spray, has no long-term damaging effects on the lungs or inner organs. It would probably even be beneficial. (Also see information in the chapter "Scientific Data and Facts".)

A great many fungi, bacteria, and germs, as well as algae, can develop in the **whirlpool, underwater massage, Jacuzzi,** or **hot-tub,** where conditions are similar. However, chemicals that attack the skin or have a strong smell shouldn't be used here either. Again, grapefruit seed extract is the appropriate antiseptic agent. Its concentration should be 10 - 20 ml (1/2 fl. oz.) of the 60% basic extract per 100 liters (22 Imp. gal., 27 US gal.) of water. This dilution corresponds to approx. 100 – 200 ppm. As you can see in the list of laboratory analyses in the Appendix of this book, great numbers of fungi, bacteria, and germs are eliminated with this concentration. However, such a high concentration might only be worthwhile in public swimming facilities where the same water is used by many visitors. People who share their private swimming pool with family members or friends and care about health and the environment might also be pleased at such a harmless and ecologically friendly means of disinfection, which will prevent algae at the same time.

Unlike chlorine, grapefruit seed extract isn't decomposed by UV rays. No harmful vapors rise and neighboring house plants aren't damaged. For people, the use of grapefruit seed extract in baths has a further advantage. Not only is possible health damage avoided—good health is promoted.

In South America, grapefruit seed extract is used in many public swimming pools. Since the extract slightly clouds the water, usually just a portion of the chlorine is replaced. However, every step in the direction of better health and a more natural lifestyle is welcome.

Public swimming pools are also known to be an "ideal" place for the transmission of athlete's foot and nail fungi which can settle on the floors of changing rooms and in showers and toilets. These floors can be wiped or sprayed with the highly effective grapefruit seed extract. A few squirts of the extract in the cleaning water are enough to prevent contagion. A higher concentration is recommended for foot baths or spray units in order to kill the athlete's foot and nail fungi more effectively and to prevent cross-contamination. We think a dosage of about 1,000 ppm would be appropriate.

Since nature offers us this effective agent in abundance, the administrators of swimming pools, spas, and hospitals, as well as medical practices and health institutes, are all asked to use this highly beneficial, and ecologically sound product.

In Drinking-Water Treatment

Clean drinking water is just as necessary for our lives as our "daily bread." For an increasing number of people today, "clean" means more than free of dirt particles and germs. Our drinking water is increasingly burdened with chemicals. Most of them reach it accidentally through the waste water from chemical waste and industrial facilities, as well as from farms However, some are intentionally added to the water, like chlorine and fluoride.

We have already reported on the very positive results of the project in Thailand where drinking water was treated with grapefruit seed extract. Adding 350 gallons of the 60% basic extract to 1 million gallons of water is enough to reduce the coli bacteria to 1 per 100 ml (3 1/2 fl. oz.). The count of these bacteria is used as a measure for the purity of drinking water, 200 coli bacteria per 100 ml are officially considered acceptable. The extract represents a highly effective, organic, and ecologically sound alternative to the customary use of chlorine. Primary benefits are the outstanding safety for the environment and for public health.

We would like to add some further thoughts on this topic. The grapefruit tree only thrives in warm countries, where the number of germs in the water is particularly high and their growth can be very rapid. Many of these are poor countries and depend on importing expensive chemicals from the industrial nations to treat their drinking water. In the rural areas, the water supply often comes from the village well. If this becomes contaminated, the whole village may become ill.

Contaminated water can be treated with a local solution, which is "growing right on the doorstep": the seed of the grapefruit tree. The use of the extract in these countries offers a number of advantages. Local production would relieve the community's budget from the expense of chemicals and save foreign currency. Manufacturing and processing the extract would create new jobs. The well-water in the villages could be disinfected in an economical and biological manner. Village communities could collect the seeds when grapefruit are eaten and make their own extract with the help of a simple coffee mill. (See the chapter "Making Grapefruit Seed Extract Yourself.") All of this is a highly remarkable prospect, isn't it?

A wonderful opportunity for providing aid to Third World countries by promoting self-help is now available. The developed nations can provide the means and knowledge to start a grapefruit seed extract production unit. For our part, we will provide the various development-aid organisations with the appropriate information when asked.

Those who desire more detailed information on biological water treatment with grapefruit seed extract can contact Knud Dencker-Jensen, consultant with a great deal of international experience (see "Addresses and Supply Sources" in the Appendix).

For Pets

While we were researching for this book, an Irish pharmaceutical manufacturer and importer told us how he came to include grapefruit seed extract in his inventory: "I had ordered several samples of the extract, and when my hunting dog got a bad fungal infection, I took advantage of the opportunity to try out the extract. Two days later, there was no trace of the fungus to be seen. The vet asked me in astonishment what I had done with the dog. When I told him about grapefruit seed extract, he pressured me until I gave him my entire supply of samples. Unfortunately, I then no longer had any myself and a new supply was far away. Now I carry grapefruit seed extract in stock and therefore always have my own supply on hand."

After this experience, he began his own investigation of the effects. When we called him four weeks later, he said: "I am positive that we are dealing with the most interesting broad spectrum therapeutic agent of the future. I don't know of any other comparable remedy, and it also appears to be superior to tea tree oil."

The healing of his hunting dog was just one of the many reports that we have received on the extract's suitability for animals, which arrived with increasing frequency. There are no plausible reasons why grapefruit seed extract, which can be used with such success for human beings, shouldn't work on animals as well. The physiology of most mammals is quite similar to our own.

Soon we also had the opportunity to try out the extract on an animal. Our cat Ananda got a stubborn fungal infection on his head. We observed it for a while, and when it continued to spread, we applied grapefruit seed extract twice a day. It took a while for the fungus to disappear completely, but the symptoms began to recede from the first treatment.

Our dog Shanty was the next "guinea pig." Almost all dogs and cats suffer from intestinal parasites and should be wormed on a regular basis. When it was once again time for Shanty to be treated, he showed all symptoms of worm infestation. We have to admit that we were delighted every time there was an opportunity for a further experiment.

However, we did not know the correct dosage for animals. So we put a capsule with 125 mg of grapefruit seed extract into his food every day for a week. He ate it without any difficulties. One day a capsule opened and the powder landed in his feeding bowl. He enjoyed his food all the same and the bowl was empty in no time. Next we tried and mixed 10 drops of the liquid extract into our cat's favorite meal, and his feeding bowl was also quickly emptied. We repeated the treatments after two weeks, and then again after four. All that we can say is that the extract was at least as effective as the chemical vermifuges.

Today we know that half of the administered amount would have been enough for our medium-sized dog, and our cat had received an even bigger overdose. Fortunately, grapefruit seed extract only leads to severe poisoning with a 4000-fold amount of the required dose, so you can hardly go wrong. We know of some pet-owners who give a preventative dose on a regular basis. It should be about half as much as for the treatment of disease.

Although it is difficult to give too large a dose of grapefruit seed extract, the optimal daily dose for animals can be determined. In order to make it easier for our readers, we have compiled a table for this purpose at the end of this chapter.

We had just finished this table when a neighbor, who had also used the extract for her dogs and cats, visited us. We proudly presented her our new work, which she glanced at sceptically. We then heard the friendly old lady's somewhat biting comment: "That's nonsense! Your table is much too complicated. Every one of my animals gets a capsule of grapefruit seed extract every day and that's it! And it works. Since I started doing this, the animals haven't been sick once. I can't start working out amounts every time—where would it end!"

In a sense, she was probably right. Since grapefruit seed extract can only lead to severe poisoning at a 4000-fold dose, her animals showed no harmful side-effects whatsoever. We later checked the figures and discovered that she had given her cats (just as we had our Ananda) about 10 to 15 times the necessary amount—without any problems. But such an approach can be expensive. If you only have one dog or cat, the cost factor may play a minor role. Things look different if you operate a dog kennel with 30 animals or have 600 sheep grazing in the meadow.

Similar to its uses for human beings, grapefruit seed extract can be applied to a broad spectrum of diseases in our four-legged friends. It has proved to be an excellent remedy for skin diseases, external injuries, and fungal infections. Internal diseases caused by bacteria, viruses, or fungi also react well to the extract. However, since an animal can't tell us what's wrong, it might be impossible to clearly diagnose the cause of an internal disease. It is well worth trying grapefruit seed extract since in most cases symptoms often subside with surprising speed.

Based on the experiences of many pet-owners, we recommend the following treatments for the individual diseases:

For **internal health disorders** due to parasites, bacteria, or fungi, put the dose specified on the list into the food. If the animal is no longer eating, try putting the less bitter powder into the drinking water.

Skin fungi or **bacterial diseases of the skin** can be sprayed with a solution. For this purpose, put 30 - 40 drops into 1 liter (35 fl. oz.) of water and pour into a spray bottle. Please make sure that it doesn't get into the animal's eyes. The extract can also be mixed with shampoo (about 10 - 40 drops, depending on the size of the animal). Shampoo the fur thoroughly with the mixture, and let it take effect for several minutes. Repeat the process after 3 days. For smaller areas and in stubborn cases, a few drops of grapefruit seed extract can be applied in full-strength or mixed with a little glycerine twice daily. However, please make sure that the animal does not lick this highly concentrated mixture and consequently damages its more delicate mouth mucous membranes.

Grapefruit seed extract can be used as a wound disinfectant for **external injuries**. It is best to use the spray described under "Skin Fungi" for this purpose. For weeping wounds, the grapefruit seed extract powder (commercially available up to now only as "grapefruit seed extract foot powder") has proved to be effective. If the animal suffers from a fungal disease in the mouth, spray diluted grapefruit seed extract (20 - 30 drops in 1 liter of water) directly into the mouth with a spray bottle—but no animal will like this.

For sick **birds**, we put a very small amount of the liquid grapefruit seed extract into the drinking water (mix well) or add a bit of extract powder to the seeds. Birds also frequently suffer from inner parasites, which can be eliminated in this simple way.

Add liquid grapefruit seed extract to the water for **fish** in the aquarium. Mix well. Start with 5 drops to 1 liter (35 fl. oz.) of water and slowly increase. The algae infestation, seen on the glass walls, should decrease as a result.

If you use ready-made grapefruit seed extract, always pay attention to the information and recommendations on the packaging. In case of doubt, consult an experienced veterinarian or animal health practitioner.

In addition, grapefruit seed extract is ideal for the disinfection of cages. You can spray or wipe them out with a solution of 20 to 30 drops of grapefruit seed extract in a bowl of water.

Feeding troughs and bowls, as well as the sleeping places of dogs and cats, can be disinfected with this solution. For washing basket pads, dog blankets, etc., put 20 drops of the extract into the last rinse.

So far we have heard of no negative reactions after using this extract on animals. If you are successful with your own experiments and would like to share your experiences for the benefit of other animals, why not publicise your results in the relevant publications or inform the animal welfare organizations about them. You may also contact the **"Grapefruit Seed Forum"** for the purpose of stimulating further research, distribution, or publication! (See "Appeal for International Cooperation" for address.)

In the Care of Livestock

On many farms, animals are given antibiotics with their feed or are drenched in order to reduce losses from disease. The use of agents against parasites is also a common occurrence. Unnatural conditions for raising livestock offer a fertile breeding ground for the transmission of diseases, particularly where animals are kept in overcrowded conditions. Chickens living in cages pick at grains that could have droppings from the other chickens stuck to them. If they have a free run, they also drink fecally contaminated rainwater that collects in little hollows in the earth. In the meadows, the animals eat grass that contains droppings from other animals.

The use of grapefruit seed extract offers many advantages. On the one hand, no harmful side effects occur. For example, the intestinal flora of the animals, which can be damaged by antibiotics, remains intact. This results in an important part of the natural defense system being maintained. The immune system of the animals is not weakened and the constitution of the animals is not additionally strained by chemicals, such as those contained in the customary vermifuges. Because of all these advantages, the chances of the animals remaining healthy in a natural manner are enormously increased. Both breeders and consumers are interested in healthy and vigorous animals. The fact that no residue is deposited in the meat of the animals is a further welcome effect. The icing on the cake is that less chemicals get into the environmental cycle.

We have received many extremely positive and enthusiastic reports about using grapefruit seed extract when raising farm animals. Pigs, cows, horses, and chickens all profit from its antibacterial, anti viral, fungicidal, and anti-parasitic effect.

The *US Department of Agriculture* in Greenport, New York, carried out a series of tests that were reported on September 7, 1982. These confirmed that in a dilution of 1:10 grapefruit seed extract was completely effective within 2 minutes against the pathogens of the dreaded **Foot-and-Mouth disease** (MKS virus), as well as the **African Swine Fever** (ASF virus). The pathogens of **Swine Vesicular Disease** (Erysipeloid) can be eliminated even with a dilution of 1:100 within 2 minutes. Since grapefruit seed extract doesn't leave undesirable deposits in tissue, its use is not subject to any limiting regulations, as is the case for antibiotics or other medications. Negative effects such as a reduction of meat quality have not been observed.

Grapefruit seed extract can be very easily mixed into the food in powder form or added to the drinking water in liquid form. The animals accept it without reservation. Higher dosages, such as that for massive worm infestation, can also be sprayed directly into the mouth. The dosage plan at the end of this chapter applies to all types of animals on a farm, at the zoo or circus, or wherever animals are kept. For acute diseases or epidemics, the dose should be doubled.

For **external diseases**, the same recommendations apply as for pets. See the last chapter on this topic. An interesting use for grapefruit seed extract would lie in the application against **hoof diseases** such as **foot rot (panaritium)**. In the damp or wet seasons particularly, sheep, goats, cattle, horses, and donkeys suffer from this problem, which can sometimes be very severe. Thanks to its antiseptic and fungicidal quality, grapefruit seed extract should be effective. It would be best to lead the animals through a shallow reservoir that has an adequate amount of the extract with as little dilution as possible. While walking through it, the hooves of the animals will be soaked with the extract. If possible, the hooves should be trimmed beforehand.

When using ready-made grapefruit seed extract for internal and external application, please always pay attention to the information and recommendations on the packaging.

In the case of notifiable diseases, the normal regulations apply, even when grapefruit seed extract is used. The extract doesn't automatically replace the advice and help of a vet or animal health practitioner—but it certainly can replace a great deal of the sometimes extremely harmful chemicals and environmental toxins that belong neither in the physiology of animals nor the biological cycles of nature.

In the course of our research for this book, we came across the agricultural consultant Knud Dencker-Jensen who has a great deal of personal experience in using the grapefruit seed extract "CitriSan®" in bio-dynamic cultivation.

He advises farmers who are converting to bio-dynamic farming and is willing to share his vast experience in using grapefruit seed extract for agricultural purposes.

However, it should be mentioned that the latest successes in raising livestock by farmers working with the bio-dynamic method cannot be attributed to the use of grapefruit seed extract alone. This method provides more appropriate conditions for raising animals and a more natural nutrition as opposed to the usual way of keeping and feeding livestock on farms. Food supplements are also fed, but they consist of such beneficial and aromatic substances as stinging nettle, fennel, woodbine, birch leaves, ash leaves, spruce needles, hazel leaves, lime leaves, willow leaves, lovage, wormwood, calendula flowers, dill, camomile, chervil, coriander, caraway, marjoram, lemon balm, peppermint, sage, yarrow flowers, thyme, hyssop, garlic, and coral calcium.

In addition to treatment and prevention of internal and external diseases, grapefruit seed extract has a further significant area of use in raising animals on farms. It can also be applied with excellent results for non-toxic **stall hygiene**. Whatever is used for successful disinfection in hospitals can be just as valuable in stalls. In earlier times, the stall walls were whitewashed once a year to disinfect them. Today, chemicals with sometimes questionable effects on health are commonly used for this purpose. Sprayed or mixed with the cleaning water, grapefruit seed extract provides a germ-free environment. In sanitary basins at the barn entrance for insemination stations or breeding compounds, the extract provides an excellent antibacterial effect without any chemical poisons clinging to shoes or hooves.

Milking facilities can be effectively disinfected with grapefruit seed extract. Since minor traces of the applied disinfectant always remain in the piping and tanks, the use of a non-toxic agent is particularly desirable here. For thorough disinfection, a concentration of a teaspoon of liquid grapefruit seed extract in 10 liters (350 fl. oz.) of water is recommended.
Here is a list to simplify dosage for internal use in animals. The guiding value is: approx. 0.5 drops of liquid grapefruit seed extract or 8 mg pulverized grapefruit seed extract should be administered per kilogram of body weight.

The therapeutically optimal daily dose of liquid grapefruit seed extract (with 33% grapefruit extractives. 20% active ingredients) and pulverized grapefruit seed extract (with 50% active ingredients) for animals with diseases caused by bacteria, viruses, parasites, and fungi or for gastrointestinal disorders would be:

Body Weight		Grapefruit Seed Extract	
		33% liquid (20%gse)	pulverized (50%gse)
1 kg		0.5 drops	approx. 8 mg
2 kg		1 drop	approx. 16 mg
5 kg		3 drops	approx. 40 mg
10 kg		6 drops	approx. 80 mg
20 kg		11 drops	approx. 145 mg
30 kg		16 drops	approx. 215 mg
40 kg		21 drops	approx. 280 mg
50 kg		27 drops	approx. 360 mg
60 kg		33 drops	approx. 440 mg
70 kg		39 drops	approx. 520 mg
80 kg approx. 1.5 ml = approx.		45 drops	approx. 600 mg
90 kg approx. 1.7 ml = approx.		51 drops	approx. 680 mg
100 kg approx. 1.9 ml = approx.		57 drops	approx. 760 mg
150 kg approx. 2.9 ml = approx.		86 drops	approx. 1.1 g
200 kg approx. 3.6 ml = approx.		108 drops	approx. 1.4 g
250 kg approx. 4.5 ml = approx.		135 drops	approx. 1.8 g
300 kg approx. 5.7 ml = approx.		171 drops	approx. 2.4 g
etc.			

In case of an acute infection the dosage may be exceeded. If using ready-made grapefruit seed extract products, always pay attention to the information on the packaging.

The therapeutically optimal daily dose of <u>pulverized grape-fruit seed extract</u> for animals with diseases caused by bacteria, viruses, parasites, and fungi or for gastrointestinal disorders would be:

For	0.4	kg body weight	approx.	1	mg
For	0.8	kg body weight	approx.	2	mg
For	1.3	kg body weight	approx.	3	mg
For	2.5	kg body weight	approx.	6	mg
For	5	kg body weight	approx.	12	mg
For	10	kg body weight	approx.	25	mg
For	20	kg body weight	approx.	50	mg
For	30	kg body weight	approx.	75	mg
For	40	kg body weight	approx.	100	mg
For	50	kg body weight	approx.	125	mg
For	60	kg body weight	approx.	150	mg
For	70	kg body weight	approx.	175	mg
For	80	kg body weight	approx.	200	mg
For	90	kg body weight	approx.	225	mg
For	100	kg body weight	approx.	250	mg
For	150	kg body weight	approx.	375	mg
For	200	kg body weight	approx.	500	mg
For	250	kg body weight	approx.	625	mg
For	300	kg body weight	approx.	750	mg
For	350	kg body weight	approx.	875	mg etc.

If using ready-made grapefruit seed extract products, always pay attention to the information on the packaging.

For Plants

One morning the sun was shining into our living room and a ray fell directly onto a plant that was one of our problem children. A large number of aphids were eating it, and so far we hadn't been able to get rid of them for any length of time. Wasn't this an invitation for a further experiment with grape-fruit seed extract? We had already successfully treated the mold on the earth of some other potted plants with a few drops of grapefruit seed extract in our watering can. But aphids?

An encyclopedia informed us about these aphids, but the book didn't say why they were so stubborn. Four different

For Plants

One morning the sun was shining into our living room and a ray fell directly onto a plant that was one of our problem children. A large number of aphids were eating it, and so far we hadn't been able to get rid of them for any length of time. Wasn't this an invitation for a further experiment with grapefruit seed extract? We had already successfully treated the mold on the earth of some other potted plants with a few drops of grapefruit seed extract in our watering can. But aphids?

An encyclopedia informed us about these aphids, but the book didn't say why they were so stubborn. Four different products from the store and two household remedies had only helped for short periods of time during the past three years. After several days or weeks, the insects had always returned and reproduced again. Finally, our experiment with grapefruit seed extract on that morning brought the desired success. We used an ordinary spray bottle and added about 30 drops of liquid extract to 1/2 liter (17.5 fl. oz.) of lukewarm water. This was shaken well so that the extract was evenly distributed in the water. On two days in a row, we sprayed the plants from all sides, not forgetting underneath the leaves, until they were soaking wet. We repeated the process two weeks later, and since then the annoying little beasts have never returned to our plants.

The application of grapefruit seed extract has also brought unexpected success with some other pests. One day we were surprised by ants invading our house, and another time a whole swarm of midges visited us at night in our bedroom. Our spray bottle was immediately put to use. We still don't know for sure why the extract was so effective—as opposed to our son Ramilan, who, observing our experiments with interest, commented: "Bodo, that's quite obvious—grapefruit burns their eyes and tastes so bitter that they prefer to beat it!" And who knows? In the end, maybe he's right

Before we begin large-scale pest-control measures, we should pause for a moment and think about how every so-called pest is assigned its very specific task in the interplay of the forces of nature. It usually only turns into a problem when there are too many of them. This in turn is frequently a sign that the balance of nature has been disturbed, and we should ask why this has occurred. However, anyone who has ever been shocked by his completely rotten tomato plants or uncovered rotting potatoes in the garden has undoubtedly attempted to intervene. With some thought he would have used a harmless agent for pest control. Grapefruit seed extract is such a biological agent: with the greatest possible spectrum of effectiveness, easy to use, ecologically tolerable, and non-toxic.

There is an enormous number of small and tiny natural organisms that can damage our plants—winegrowers, fruitgrowers, farmers, and gardeners can tell us a thing or two about them. The trend today is to intervene as gently as possible without immediately exterminating the entire range of microorganisms above and below the soil.

In order to control pests in a meaningful way, it is necessary to be familiar with the biological life cycles of the individual insects, bacteria, and fungal cultures. On the basis of this knowledge, you could reduce the application of pest-control agents to a minimum. You would now use the agents in a very specific and therefore extremely effective manner, saving a great deal of time and money. But who knows that to avoid strawberry-fruit rot (also called botrytis), it is necessary to spray twice during the period between first blossoming and the beginning of the second fruit ripening, at intervals of 14 days, or that seed treatment is necessary to combat tomato-stem rot?. For our northern latitudes alone, it would be necessary to study the life and reproduction cycles of 140 so-called pests, together with their specific food, development, and wintering characteristics.

For a large number of plant diseases, grapefruit seed extract could be worth considering as a biologically meaningful alternative to the usual preparations. Where aphids are concerned, we can only report on our own successful experiments. Yet, the extract has already proved itself effective in cases of rot and fungal infestation. We have heard of success with spraying potatoes, leeks, and carrots.

Many plant diseases are caused by putrefactive agents and fungi. Where damage is caused by the red spider mite in hops, collar rot in trees, cabbage mildew in the seedbed, potato-vine rot, cucumber scab, pear scurf, lettuce rot, celery-leaf blotch, spinach mildew, leaf spot in beans and peas, snow mold in rye and wheat, wheat bunt, heart or dry rot in beets, tobacco wildfire, fruit-tree cancer, peach leaf curl, downy mildew in currants and gooseberries, etc. - grapefruit seed extract would be an appropriate measure for pest control in all of these cases. If we consider the above-mentioned life cycles and take specific action, we would have a pest-control program that would be ideal. A thick book could be written on this topic alone. However, it is probably just a matter of time until a helpful guide is published that will tell us how, when, and why this fungus or that disease can be controlled with grapefruit seed extract.

Industry will certainly soon manufacture and offer special, easy-to-use preparations that include grapefruit seed extract and are also suitable for a large-scale application in agriculture, fruitgrowing, winegrowing, and gardening. The occasional inquiries on the part of future users directed to the researchers and producers may contribute to advancing these products. The impetus in this direction will certainly come from farmers who work with organic or bio-dynamic methods.

Just as we were writing this, we received an inquiry from German environmentalists working on an experiment to try and heal elm trees that have Dutch Elm Disease. This problem kills many elm trees and is now widespread in Europe. Biologists have recognized that a fungus plays an active role in the course of the disease. This means that the chances for success should be quite good. It is still too early to report on results, but why not risk such an experiment? In the not too distant future, we could possibly have more good news to spread.

We encourage you to publicize experiments and practical successes with the application of grapefruit seed extract for plants in the relevant publications or also report on them to the **"Grapefruit Seed Forum"** for further research, dissemination, or publication (see "Appeal for International Co-operation" for address)!

When using the corresponding ready-made products, please pay attention to their respective dosages and procedures.

Common measuring values used in this book can be found in the table on page 112.

Making Grapefruit Seed Extract Yourself

One November day in 1995, a violent hurricane swept across the Southwest of Ireland. Living on the Atlantic coast, we receive the full force of storms like this. Shortly after the storm started, the electricity supply was cut off, the telephone and fax ceased to function, and our work at the computer was put on ice. So, making the best of the situation, we sat close together in front of the warming fire and talked about the topic that had been occupying us for months—grapefruit seed extract. It suddenly occurred to us that we had given away our last bottle of extract to a German photographer who had visited us a few days ago. Shalila asked casually: "Do you think we could make grapefruit seed extract ourselves?" - "Let's try it," was Bodo's response since we had plenty of grapefruits in the house.

So, first there was some delicious grapefruit juice, and we carefully picked out the seeds. We then tried to somehow squeeze out the seeds, but that was easier said than done. Bodo tried to do this with everything he could find in the kitchen, the workshop, and even the garden shed. All that he achieved was a huge mess when he tried to squeeze the contents out of the slippery seeds with a hammer or any other tool. Our little son Ramilan had lots of fun watching him, especially when the seeds squirted in all directions and his father grumbled to himself in annoyance. His attempt to crush the seeds in a mortar also failed miserably.

Second attempt: We had a better idea. Why not simply grind the grapefruit seeds? Although we couldn't use our electric mill because of the power cut, we still had an old hand mill in the cupboard that ought to do the job just as well. However, we soon found that the fresh seeds completely clogged the mill and stuck to the grinding surfaces. After just a few rotations, it broke down—and the same thing would have happened to our larger electric mill.

Third attempt: It became clear to us that the seeds had to be dried before grinding them, which we should have thought of in the first place. So we put the seeds on a tray and set it as close to the fire as possible (the oven was useless because of the power cut). Now we had to be sure that the seeds didn't get too hot since we didn't want the grapefruit seeds roasted. just well dried. When our oven was working again, we found that a temperature between 104 and 112 degrees F. is adequate. A drying kiln could also be used for this purpose. Naturally the sun will also dry the seeds when the weather is good.

After drying, the grapefruit seeds were shrivelled up and almost as light as paper. Since our mill was clogged and we couldn't clean it because there was not enough light, we had to postpone further processing. Here is the result of our later attempt.

When the seeds are ground, we find two different components: a fine flour, from the ground kernels, and the hulls of the seeds, which look something like the husks when grain is ground. In order to separate the two components, we shook everything through a tightly meshed household sieve, which gave us a fine grapefruit seed powder. We were very proud of our successful attempt. Later we compared the color and taste of our powder with that of the ready-made capsules, and couldn't discover any difference.

The procedure is quite simple, even if it does take some time. However, where do you get the many grapefruit seeds necessary to fill even a little bottle? If you have to buy all the grapefruits it will be uneconomic. Perhaps you could persuade your friends and relatives to start collecting all their grapefruit seeds for you. Maybe you can find a juice bar that usually throws the seeds away.

You could possibly get a large enough amount together, but caution is required. Storing the moist seeds for a period of time could cause mold on the outer hull of the seed, particularly if they are closely packed in a container without enough air circulating. However, this phenomenon shows that the active fungicidal ingredients are inside the grapefruit seed and not in the outer hull.

If you want to make it easy for yourself, you can simply chew the seeds after removing the outer hull. We've heard of various successful experiments of this type. However, in order to make the active ingredients sufficiently accessible, the seeds must be chewed very thoroughly.

We are not in a position to say whether taking home-made powder or chewing the seeds will be as effective as the commercial product. This is due to the additional processes which take place when commercially manufactured. These processes have not been disclosed to us by the manufacturers.

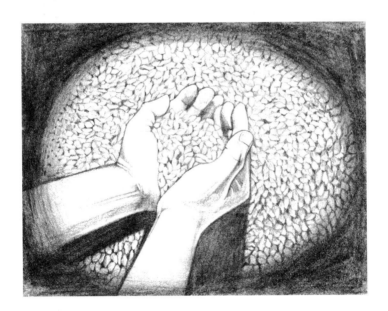

Scientific Data and Facts

PRODUCTION

Commercially produced grapefruit seed extract is made by a bio-technical process from grapefruit seeds and pulp. (See the chapter "A Tree Called "Citrus Paradisi"")

COMPONENTS

The grapefruit seed extract primarily contains bioflavinoids and glycosides in the form of naringin (naringenin rutinosid), isosacuranetin (didymin), neohesperidin, hesperidin, dihydrocampherol glycoside, poncirin, quercetin glycoside, campherol glycoside, apigenin rutinoside, rhoifolin, heptamothoxyflavone, nobiletin, as well as several proteins.

PROPERTIES

Grapefruit seed extract has the ability to interfere with the normal processes of decay by inhibiting and killing the microorganisms that are the root cause. It de-activates pathogens and is capable of dealing with many parasites. The extract has a very low level of toxicity to humans and other mammals and does not damage the environment. This has been proven in tests and laboratory experiments carried out, independently of each other, in several countries. These experiments included tests on bacterial, viral, and fungal cultures and parasites, as well as on animals and human beings. They showed that the extract is highly effective against a broad spectrum of germs, such as *Staphylococcus*, *Streptococcus*, *Salmonella*, *E. coli*, *Pseudomonas*, *Lactobacillus*, *Klebsiella*, *Shigella*, *Legionella*, *Chlamydia*, *Helicobacter*, *Herpes*, and strongly inhibits fungi and yeasts. The results of these experiments can be found in the laboratory analyses. The extract has a characteristic citrus odor that is no longer perceptible in the concentrations normally used. Vegetable glycerine is generally used as a base for the liquid extract and this further enriches the flavone complex of citrus fruit.

MODE OF ACTIVITY

According to studies, the antimicrobial activity of grapefruit seed extract appears to develop in the cytoplasmic membrane of the micro-organisms. The active ingredients of the extract disorganise the cytoplasmic membrane, thereby preventing the uptake of amino acids. At the same time, there is a leakage of the cellular contents with low molecular weight through the cytoplasmic membrane. The pathogen is inactivated and dies. The time required for this is generally shorter than that of most comparable preparations for eliminating micro-organisms. Newer studies on selected micro-organisms confirm two primary effects: (1) an alteration of the cell membrane with inhibition of cellular respiration and (2) a dose-dependent inhibition of cellular respiration. Heating or freezing the extract does not destroy its effectiveness.

TOXIC SAFETY

No health dangers are known for grapefruit seed extract when used properly. Under normal use, the extract is neither toxic nor a primary skin irritant. To date, there are no known cases of poisoning. In various animal experiments carried out by independent laboratories, at least 5 g of 50% grapefruit seed extract per kilogram of body weight had to be administered before a lethal poisoning occurred in some cases. On the basis of these results;

for 60 kilograms of body weight, at least 300 g
for 70 kilograms of body weight, at least 350 g
for 80 kilograms of body weight, at least 400 g
for 90 kilograms of body weight, at least 450 g

of grapefruit seed extract (with a 50% concentration of active substances) would have to be administered orally in order to produce severe poisoning. This corresponds to approximately 4000 times the amount of a normal dose of 0.1 gram of grapefruit seed extract powder or about 12 drops of the liquid form. This clearly shows how safe the extract is in normal use.

LABORATORY EXPERIMENTS ON LIVING SUBJECTS

We are against animal experiments that involve any kind of cruelty. However, we have received the results of some tests (prescribed by law in the USA) that we present here for the sake of completeness:

In a test to determine acute toxicity, 10 rats were administered a single dose of 5000 mg/kg of body weight. Two days later, one of the rats showed signs of lethargy. After three days, one of the rats died. The others showed no signs of poisoning up to the end of the 14-day test. The test report concludes with the statement that the average lethal dose (LD50) of grapefruit seed extract lies above the value of 5000 mg/kg of body weight. This value was confirmed by further tests. On the basis of these tests, grapefruit seed extract has been classified as generally non-toxic.

Three further tests were carried out to determine the chronic toxicity. In a 12-month test, adult rats were given grapefruit seed extract with their food every day. A daily dose of 2900 mg/kg body weight was necessary before the rats died. For human beings, this means that a person weighing 80 kg would have to drink about 580 ml of a customary grapefruit seed extract every day for twelve months before the extract would have a fatal effect. In another 12-month test on new-born rats, three of the animals died after a daily dose of 400 mg of grapefruit seed extract per kilogram of body weight had been administered. A daily dose averaging 1992 mg/kg of body weight over a 24-month period led to death in adult rats and guinea pigs.

A **two-year skin cancer test** with Citricidal® on rats and mice showed no type of damage on the skin or within the inner organ systems.

There is considered to be no general **cancer risk** through Citricidal®.

An allergy skin test on humans showed no irritation or sensitization at a dilution of 1% and 2% (this corresponds to about 50 or 100 drops in a glass of water). A solution of 3% (150 drops in a glass of water), produced slight irritation for people with allergies.

If the full-strength extract gets into the eyes, a severe irritation with slight corneal iris injury occurs. Concentrations of 0.5%, 1%, and 2% cause irritation and moderate reddening.

A further test researched the **effects of long-term inhalation** of Citricidal® through the lungs in a closed chamber. The test ran for 90 days, 5 days a week, and 8 hours a day. The concentration of the grapefruit seed extract as a test substance consisted of 100 - 150 mg per cubic meter of air. No negative health effects were observed.

FIRST-AID MEASURES

In case of an emergency: if grapefruit seed extract gets into the eyes, wash them out immediately with plenty of water (warm if possible) and consult a doctor, if necessary.

After an excessive ingestion of grapefruit seed extract, drink plenty of water. Up to 3 teaspoons of psyllium husks (Indian fleawort seed hulls) with 1 glass of water or up to 6 psyllium capsules can also be taken. Consult a doctor, if necessary.

Never take grapefruit seed extract full-strength or in an undiluted form!

If there are discernible, undesirable skin irritations, wash off the extract with plenty of water.

ENVIRONMENTAL ASPECTS

Researchers from an American laboratory have confirmed that no damage to the environment is to be expected from the release of grapefruit seed extract. A 5-year study conducted in the USA has shown that the extract doesn't accumulate in the soil. Concentrations of 50 - 100 ppm* of the 60% basic extract were sprayed onto sand and clay soil. After one hour, a concentration of less than 1:1 billion of the sprayed extract remained detectable with a gas chromatograph. The extract is completely decomposed after 24 hours at an administration concentration of 50 ppm* and after 8 days at an administration concentration of 100 ppm*. Grapefruit seed extract has accordingly been classified in the USA as *non-ecotoxic.*

According to current estimations, no additional cultivation areas will be required for grapefruit seed extract, even if there is a substantial increase in demand, since only a fraction of the seed material is used for further processing. For political reasons relating to work and social circumstances, as well as transportation and environmental considerations, the extract should

---

* ppm = parts per million = 1 per 1,000,000

be manufactured in those countries where grapefruit is culti-vated, harvested, and made into juice. This would create fur-ther, sorely needed jobs in some of the Third World nations.

We would therefore like to suggest that European manu-facturers and processors of grapefruit seed extract develop their sources of raw material as far as possible in the countries bor-dering the Mediterranean instead of importing the extract from the USA or South America. The Asian countries should satisfy their needs for grapefruit seed material from Southeast Asia, the Australians in Australia, and the African countries in Africa. There are no plausible reasons for transporting this valuable raw material halfway around the world.

SPECTRUM OF APPLICATIONS

In addition to curing and preventing diseases in humans and animals, grapefruit seed extract has been successfully used for sterilization, demycotization, and preservation. Chicken, fish, shellfish, nuts, vegetables, fruit, and drinking water have all been treated in this way. There are many agricultural, horti-cultural, industrial, and domestic uses. The extract is tolerant to acids, and therefore used in acidic biological cleaning agents. It is highly compatible with non-ionic agents, ascorbic acid, acetic acid, citric acid, sodium acetate, potassium hydroxide, borax, sodium sulfate, and sodium carbonate. Because of its biological origin, grapefruit seed extract is particularly popular in natural cosmetics. The extract can easily be worked into preparations during the aqueous phase and is also soluble in butylene alcohol, alcohol, and some other organic solvents. The extract has good mixing qualities in application concen-trations of 0.2% - 1% and is compatible with the most commonly used inactive ingredients, including triton X and isopropyl alcohol. (As already mentioned elsewhere, isopropyl alcohol participates substantially in the development of cancer accord-ing to Dr. Hulda Regehr Clark's research. We therefore do not recommend its use.)

STORAGE

Grapefruit seed extract should be stored safely away from children. It should be labelled, tightly closed, and kept in a dark and cool place. It stays fresh and suitable for processing over long periods of time. Rotting or infestation with germs or mold is almost impossible. When handling large amounts, wear safety goggles as a precautionary measure.

TEST OF A BRAND PRODUCT

Citricidal® from the USA is the brand name of a standardized extract of 60% grapefruit seeds (with the addition of grapefruit cell membrane) in an aqueous, vegetable glycerine solution (40%) without metallic ingredients, as a preservative and broad spectrum antiseptic with strong bactericidal and fungicidal properties. (Citricidal® sold in the U.K. and Ireland contains 33% extract and 67% glycerine.)

Citricidal® has been approved by the CTFA (USA) and is labelled as "Grapefruit Seed Extract." Citricidal® has been listed in the USA as "GRAS" (Generally Recognized as Safe) in the Code of Federal Regulations under Number 21 CFR 182.20. The FDA has approved Citricidal® for cosmetic preparations with the CRMS No. R 0013982. In addition, Citricidal® has also been approved by the FDA for the treatment (disinfection) of foods. Citricidal® received the CAS No. 90045-43-5. Citricidal® is non-ecotoxic and does not accumulate in the soil.

Chemical and Physical Properties
of Citricidal®

Chemical Description:	Diphenol hydroxybenzene complex
Appearance:	Liquid/heavy viscous
Color (Gardner):	2, Lemon Yellow
Odor:	Mild citrus
Specific Gravity (77° F):	1.110
Density (lbs./gal.):	9.5
pH (77° F):	2.0 - 3.0
Molecular Weight:	565
Flash:	292° F
Viscosity (Centistoke):	134.91
Solubility (Solvent):	Water, alcohol, and organic solvents

Laboratory Analyses

Analyses on the effectiveness of grapefruit seed extract for bacteria, viruses, and fungi were conducted from 1991 to 1993 by:

Bio/Chem Research Inc., Lakeport, CA, USA
Valley Microbiology Services, Palo Alto, CA, USA
Bio-Research Laboratories, Redmond, WA, USA
British Columbia Research Corp., Vancouver, B.C., Canada
Northview Pacific Laboratories, Inc., Berkeley, CA, USA

The studies were carried out with the basic extract (undiluted Citricidal®) which contains 60% grapefruit seed extract and 40% glycerine (veg. U.S.P., which is used in the manufactoring process). The agent is supplied by the manufacturer in this concentration and only used by doctors in the USA. The liquid extract on the open market in the USA and in Europe (incl. Citricidal®) usually contain 1 part of the basic extract, to which 2 parts of glycerine or water are added. This dilution is normally labelled as 33% active ingredients, grapefruit seed extract or Citricidal. In actual fact it contains only 20% grapefruit extractives, since the basic extract already contains 40% of glycerine.

In the following laboratory studies, the respective minimum inhibitory concentration of Citricidal® from the USA is shown, stated in millionth fractions (MIC = ppm = parts per million).

No. of drops required in a cup of water (200 ml) for given strenghts

Strenght in ppm	100% basic extract (60%)	33% extract (20%)
333	2 drops	6 drops
666	4 drops	12 drops
1000	6 drops	18 drops
2000	12 drops	36 drops

Citricidal®* Minimum Inhibitory Concentration In Vitro (MIC)*

Gram-Positive Bacteria	Source	Strain No.:	MIC (ppm):
Bacillus subtilis	NCTC	8236	2
Bacillus megatherium	A	-	60
Bacillus cereus	A	-	60
Bacillus cereus var. mycoides	A	-	60
Clostridium botulinum	NCTC	3805	60
Clostridium tetani	NCTC	9571	60
Corynebacterium	ATCC	6919	60
Corynebacterium diphtheriae	ATCC	6917	60
Corynebacterium diphtheriae	NCTC	3984	60
Corynebacterium diphtheriae	A	-	60
Corynebacterium minutissium	ATCC	6501	100
Diplococcus pneumoniae	NTCT	7465	60
Giardia lamblia	ATTC	30957	1000
Lactobacillus arabinosus	CITM	707	66
Lactobacillus arabinosus	ATCC	8014	66
Lactobacillus casei	CITM	707	100
Listeria monocytogenes	ATCC	15313	20
Mycobacterium tuberculosis	A	-	2000
Mycobacterium smegmatis	NCTC	8152	20
Mycobacterium phelei	A	-	6
Sarcina lutea	NCTC	196	60
Sarcinaureae	ATCC	6473	2
Staphylococcus aureas	NCTC	7447	2
Staphylococcus aureas	NCTC	4163	2
Staphylococcus aureas	NCTC	6571	6
Staphylococcus aureas	NCTC	6966	2
Staphylococcus aureas	ATCC	13709	2
Staphylococcus aureas	ATCC	6538	2
Staphylococcus albus	NCTC	7292	2
Staphylococcus albus	C.-G.	-	6
Streptococcus agalactiae	NCTC	8181	60
Streptococcus haemoyticus A	A	-	20
Streptococcus faecalis	NCTC	8619	200
Streptococcus faecalis	ATCC	10541	60
Streptococcus pyogenes	NCTC	8322	60
Streptococcus viridans	-	-	20

Gram-Negative Bacteria:	Source	Strain No.:	MIC (ppm):
Aerobacter aerogenes	CTTM	413	20
Alcalingenes faecalis	A	-	2000
Brucella intermedia	A	-	2
Brucella abortus	NCTC	8226	2
Brucella melitensis	A	-	2
Brucella suis	A	-	2
Cloaca cloacae	NCTC	8155	6
Escherichia coli	NCTC	86	2
Escherichia coli	ATCC	9663	6
Escherichia coli	ATCC	11229	16
Escherichia coli	NCTC	9001	6
Haemophilus influenzae	A	-	660
Klebsiella edwardsii	NCTC	7242	6
Klebsiella aerogenes	NCTC	8172	6
Klebsiella pneumoniae	ATCC	4352	6
Legionella pneumoniae	isolate	-	200
Loefflerella mallei	NCTC	9674	6
Loefflerella pseudomallei	NCIB	10230	20
Moraxella duplex	A	-	2
Moraxella glucidolytica	A	-	6
Neisseria catarrhalis	NCTC	3622	660
Pseudomonas aeruginosa	ATCC	15442	250
Pseudomonas capacia	C-175	-	5000
Pasteurella septica	NCTC	948	2
Pasteurella pseudotuberculosis	C.-G.	-	200
Proteus vulgaris	NCTC	8313	2
Proteus mirabilis	A	-	6
Pseudomonas aeruginosa	NTCT	1999	2000
Pseudomonas aeruginosa	ATCC	12055	20.000
Pseudomonas fluorescens	NCTC	4755	2000
Salmonella choleraesuis	-	-	50
Salmonella choleraesuis	ATCC	10708	660
Salmonella enteritidis	A	-	6
Salmonella gallinarum	-	-	50
Salmonella typhimurium	NCTC	5710	6
Salmonella typhi	NCTC	8384	6
Salmonella paratyphi A	NCTC	5322	6
Salmonella paratyphi B	NCTC	3176	6

Salmonella pullorum	ATCC	9120	6
Serratia marcescens	A	-	2000
Shigella flexneri	NCTC	8192	6
Shigella sonnei	NCTC	7240	3
Shigella dysenteriae	NCTC	2249	2
Vibrio cholerae	A	-	200
Vibrio eltor	NCTC	8457	200

Fungi and Yeasts:	Source	Strain No.:	MIC (ppm):
Aspergillus niger	ATCC	6275	600
Aspergillus flavis	ATCC	9643	78
Aspergillus fumigatus	ATCC	9197	200
Aureobasidium pullulans	ATCC	9348	10
Candida albicans	A	-	60
Candida albicans	ATCC	10259	60
Chaetomium globosum	ATCC	6205	3
Epidermophyton floccosum	ATCC	10227	200
Keratinomyces ajelloi	A	-	200
Monilia albicans	-	-	10
Penicillium roqueforti	ATCC	6989	5
Saccharomyces cerevisiae	-	-	60
Trichophyton mentagrophytes	ATCC	9533	20
Trichophyton rubrum	A	-	200
Trichophyton tonsurans	A	-	200

FURTHER EFFICACY STUDIES

The effectiveness of grapefruit seed extract has also been proved on the following micro-organisms in laboratory experiments at various institutes.*

Alphabetic List:

Agaricus bisporus
Aspergillus crysstallilnus
Aspergillus fischeri
Aspergillus flavus
Aspergillus oryzae
Aspergillus parasiticus
Aspergillus terreus
Campylobacter jejuni
Chaetomium globosum
Chlamydia trachomatis
Entamoeba histolytica
Enterobacter sp.
Fusarium oxysporum

Fusarium sambucinum
Fusariumsp. tuberosi
Giardia lamblia
Helicobacter pylori
Herpes Simplex Virus, Type 1
Influenza A_2 Virus
Lactobacillus pentoaceticus
Measles Virus Morbillium
Penicillium funiculosum
Pullularia pullulans
Scerotinia laxa
Trichomonas vaginalis
Trichophyton interdigitalis

In another efficacy study** in the USA, a grapefruit seed extract by the name of ParaMycrocidin® with a concentration of 0.001% - 2% was tested on 794 bacterial strains and 93 fungal strains. In the process, the effectiveness of this remedy was proved for 249 Staph. aureus, 86 Streptococcus sp., 232 Enterococcus sp., 77 Enterobacter sp., 86 E. Coli sp., 22 Klebsiella sp., 18 Proteus sp., 71 yeast fungal, and 22 mold fungal strains.

---

* The detailed test data was unfortunately not available at the time of printing. Furthermore, not every laboratory/manufacturer made its test results available. Our research sometimes turned into complicated detective work since some manufacturers thought that we were possibly industrial spies for a giant chemical company.

** Ionescu, G./Kiehl, R./ Wichmann-Kunz, F./ Williams, Ch./Bäuml, L./ Levine, S.: "Oral Citrus Seed Extract in Atopic Eczema: In Vitro and In Vivo Studies on Intestinal Microflora," Journal of Orthomolecular Medicine, Volume 5, No. 3, USA, 1990.

Study on the Relative Efficacy
of Grapefruit Seed Extract in Comparison to Other
Common Antimicrobial Active Ingredients

The minimal bacteriostatic concentration study is a microbial study that has been used to compare the relative efficacy of grapefruit seed extract (Citricidal®) with other antimicrobial substances. The study demonstrated that grapefruit seed extract (Citricidal®) is 10 times to 100 times more effective against the organisms tested in the study than the other test substances.

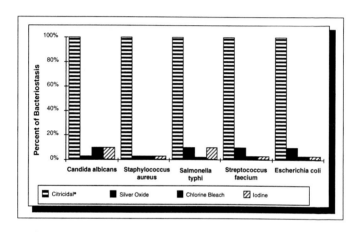

Study on the Preservation Efficacy
of Grapefruit Seed Extract

The study on the efficacy of preservation evaluated the ability of products to resist microbial attacks. The study was specially designed to determine whether a product is protected from micro-organisms that could effect a qualitative or structural change in the product. The study showed that 0.2% methylparaben took a week to significantly reduce the micro-organisms in the product while 0.2% Citricidal® (grapefruit seed extract) achieved this level in just one day.

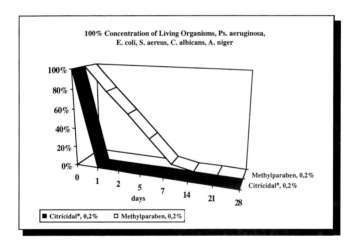

General Information for Clarification and Simplification of the Dosage for Grapefruit Seed Extract in Daily Practice

1 ppm	= 1 part per million
1 ml	= 1 milliliter, one-thousandth of a liter
1 l	= 1 liter, one thousand milliliters, 35 fl. oz.
1 fl. oz.	= 29 ml (approx.)
1 pint	= 16 fl. oz. (US), 20 fl. oz. (Imp.)
1 mg	= 1 milligram, one-thousandth of a gram (0.001 g)
1 g	= 1 gram = the weight of 1 ml of water at STP
1 kg	= 1 kilogram, one thousand grams
1 oz.	= 28.4 grams
1 lb.	= 16 oz. = 454 grams

Liquid Grapefruit Seed Extract:

1 teaspoon   corresponds to approx. 5 ml
              = approx.   75 drops
1 tablespoon corresponds to approx. 10 ml
              = approx. 150 drops
1 ml   corresponds to approx. 15 drops

Grapefruit Seed Extract Powder:

100 mg   corresponds to approx. 10 - 12 drops of liquid
= (0.1 g)   grapefruit seed extract (such as Citricidal®)

Additional Ideas and Product Suggestions

We encourage everyone to use products which are environmentally friendly and biologically effective and so we would like to make some suggestions for additional uses of grapefruit seed extract. Some of these are currently being tested and new products will soon be available to the public.

We ask all those who are involved in the production and sale of similar items and materials to use their imagination to discover new uses and consider using grapefruit seed extract wherever possible. Thank-you.*

Grapefruit seed extract, with its antibacterial, anti-fungal, anti-viral and anti-parasitic properties, can be used as an active ingredient and / or preservative in the following:

baby care products such as
- powders
- creams
- lotions
- disposable diapers

personal hygiene products such as
- soaps and hand-cleaners
- shower gels
- medical shampoos
- shaving foam, shaving creams and after-shave lotions
- bubble baths
- face and body creams
- deodorant sticks and sprays
- suntan lotions and creams
- acne creams and lotions
- cotton buds

---

* Some of the possibilities and products listed here have already been put into practice while we were writing this book. Others are currently in the trial phase.

dental care products such as
- toothpastes
- mouth washes and mouth sprays
- chewing gum for prevention of caries and gingivitis
- effervescent tablets for cleaning of dentures
- wooden toothpicks
- dental floss
- disinfectant in dental practices
- tooth fillings

feminine hygiene products such as
- panty liners
- sanitary pads
- tampons
- feminine douches
- vaginal sprays and gels

cosmetic articles such as
- make up
- face creams and lotions
- cleansing lotions
- lipsticks (for prevention and treatment of *Herpes simplex*)
- nail varnish and polish (for prevention of nail fungus)

medical products such as
- creams for wounds
- plasters, wound dressings, bandages
- ready-made swabs
- skin disinfectants for use before surgical operations
- antiseptic lubricants and active disinfectant in condoms and surgical gloves
- medical/clinical hand-washing gels
- drops, lozenges and syrups for coughs, colds, sore throats, laryngitis, tonsillitis and pharyngeal catarrh
- nasal spray
- ear drops
- vaginal suppositories for treatment of ovarian cysts
- sprays, creams and powders for treatment of athlete's foot and other fungal infections
- remedies for nail fungus

hygiene products for use in domestic, commercial and municipal buildings and facilities such as
- household cleaners
- dishwasher and washing machine detergent
- carpet cleaner
- sprays and solutions for general hygiene in medical practices, hospitals, day-care centers, care for the aged and the sick, etc.
- disinfectants for medical equipment and instruments
- foot-disinfection units in public swimming facilities
- cleaning agents for swimming facilities, saunas, fitness studios, and solariums
- room sprays
- solution in air-conditioning systems, humidifiers and dehumidifiers
- fungicide for treating mold in damp rooms

products for the care of domestic and farm animals such as
- medical shampoos and sprays
- vermifuges
- animal hoof treatments
- antiseptic treatments for wounds
- disinfectants for kennels, stalls, stables
- water treatment in fish farms and aquaria

products for horticultural use such as
- agents to keep cut flowers fresh
- sprays for plant pests on house plants
- fungicide and pesticide sprays
- seed preservative against rot and mold
- application in forestry against various tree diseases and infestation with molds and parasites

products for disinfection and preservation in the food industry such as
- preservatives for fresh foods such as grains, fruit, vegetables, fish and meat
- preservatives for processed foods and drinks
- disinfectant for milking facilities
- disinfectants for food processing and filling facilities as well as cleaning reusable bottles and jars

115

products for additional uses such as
- water treatment, both personal and municipal
- wood preservatives
- bactericide and fungicide in carpets, fabrics and other materials.

Our prognosis is that by the year 2000 many of these possibilities will have been realized. Shall we bet on it?

Every problem
goes through three stages until it is recognized:
first it is made fun of
second it is contested
third it is considered obvious.

ARTHUR SCHOPENHAUER (1788-1860)

Appeal for International Cooperation

If each of us wanted to help another person
Then all of us would already be helped

BARONESS MARIE VON EBNER-ESCHENBACH (1830-1916)
FROM "APHORISMS"

It is likely that many readers of this book will have their own experiences with grapefruit seed extract in the course of the next weeks and months, allowing them to confirm the effect of this interesting extract. More than a few people have a natural tendency to experiment and will attempt to use grapefruit seed extract in further areas of their life, just as we did. We strongly advise you to be very careful and circumspect. Your own health and well-being should always have top priority! Above all, we are *not* calling for these types of experiments.

However, "living-room experiments" can lead to the discovery of many new areas of application for grapefruit seed extract. Doctors, naturopaths, nurses, midwives, druggists, pharmacists, chiropodists, cosmeticians, health consultants, physiotherapists, chemists, animal-keepers and livestock-breeders, farmers and gardeners who are inspired by our book to use grapefruit seed extract themselves will come across further interesting areas of application and collect a wealth of their own experiences. At this point, we would like to suggest that these experiences and knowledge be made available to the general public to inspire further research.

For this purpose, we have created a **"Grapefruit Seed Forum"** that accepts, catalogs, and evaluates experiences with and observations about grapefruit seed extract. It will pass these on to responsible scientists, practitioners, and manufacturers. If these experiences are confirmed by scientific findings or by a convincing number of similar reports, they will be passed on to such media as the press, radio, television, and Internet for the benefit of all. Please send information about interesting

117

experiences, findings, and observations with grapefruit seed extract or related products to:

GRAPEFRUIT SEED FORUM
Ardnatrush, Vale Cove
Glengarriff, Co. Cork
Ireland
Fax 027/6 31 28

If possible, please send the information in German, English, Dutch, or French—and warmest thanks in the name of all those who will benefit from these findings in the future!!!

We would encourage you to pass on any personal experiences with and knowledge about grapefruit seed extract. You may wish to share this in the form of articles and letters to the editor of any relevant publications or contributions to discussion groups and television and radio programs.

A request: Please do not write to us with specific medical enquiries like "Does grapefruit seed extract work in this special case or not?" In order to give advice, an accurate diagnosis and full examination of the affected person, together with any case history, is necessary. It is therefore more appropriate and worthwhile to consult an experienced doctor or naturopath.

Concluding Observations

Nature creates nothing without significance.
ARISTOTLE (384 - 322 B.C.)

If you have read this book, you will probably agree with us that the seed of the grapefruit is a very special gift of nature, which fascinates and amazes with its many talents. Researchers and scientists have only just begun their studies, and we will certainly hear of more interesting discoveries in the future.

Yet, the findings presented in this book should not cause us to make declared enemies of bacteria, viruses, fungi, and other micro-organisms or become phobic about them, since everything in Creation is known to have its purpose. It may be that certain mechanisms that were originally in balance have lost their equilibrium. However, we human beings are usually the cause of such disturbances. It is important to learn for the future and develop a much greater sensitivity when dealing with the forces of nature. Fortunately, it also appears that a change in our way of thinking has begun on a wide front.

At this point, we would like to return to the thought that we expressed at the beginning—that we are required to learn or develop whenever we are ill. Every illness provides an opportunity of directing our attention towards unfulfilled or neglected areas of our consciousness and can lead us to our own further development. From this perspective, illness is not evil or a perversity of nature but a meaningful challenge for our individual destiny. It becomes an exhortation for us to grow, to accept, and to integrate those parts of ourselves that we have suppressed and separated from the wholeness of existence. True healing is always connected with the growth of an individual and an increase in perception. This cannot be replaced by some new remedy—not even the beneficial extract from the grapefruit seed.

This perception does not rule out the possibility for us to seek and accept help on the material level since our existence also takes place on the material plane. It is important to understand that we exist on many levels and need to find an equilibrium which will bring all levels back into a balanced, holistic state. This equilibrium will contain both spirit and matter, heaven and earth, mind and emotions, masculine and feminine within it.

In this sense, with respect, gratitude, and joy we should honor the grace of nature that gives us blessings like the miracle in the seed of the grapefruit, which can improve the quality of our life and well-being in such a simple way.

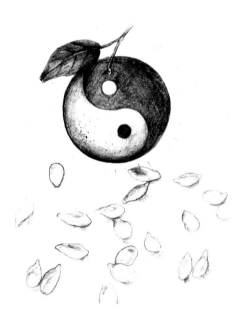

Acknowledgements

For their wonderful help and support in the creation of this book, from the bottom of our hearts we would like to thank:

Utella Hackmann (Ireland), who brought order to the office time and again, corrected texts, and contributed many useful ideas

Alan Dare (Ireland), who introduced us to his knowledge of and experiences with grapefruit seed extract

Julia Kemp (Ireland), for her help and suggestions.

Mike Tanner (Ireland), for his valuable work with the American edition.

Knud Dencker-Jensen (Denmark), who we thank very much for his openness regarding his experiences with grapefruit seed extract in agriculture

Celia and Brian Wright (Great Britain) for their courageous pioneer work in the international dissemination of knowledge about grapefruit seed extract

Dixie Shipp (USA) for her great support in our research in the USA and Asia

Jürgen Kolb (Germany) for his international research on the Internet and his computer graphics

Alois Hanslian (Germany), the artist, for his attractive illustrations in the book

Racky Baginski (Germany), Bodo's brother, for his expert advice in the agricultural field

Hans Jürgen Colombara (Germany) and
Norbert Harmuth (Germany), the pharmacists, for their friendly support

Ramilan, our son, who was so patient and understanding while we were busy with this book

Monika and **Wolfgang Jünemann** (Germany), our active and determined publishers, who have been willing to engage in new, courageous deeds of journalistic trailblazing time and again.

We would also like to thank all of our friends and readers who may take part in the international dissemination of knowledge about the various effects and uses for grapefruit seed extract. By so doing, they will give active support to a healthier and more natural way of life, as well as the recovery of nature.

The Authors

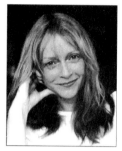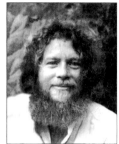

Shalila Sharamon, born on July 24, 1948, was trained as a meditation teacher in 1972. She established and directed several meditation centers. In 1980, she began to study astrology and since 1992 has specialised in Jyotish, the astrology of India. She combines her astrological knowledge with holistic personal and health counselling. While traveling through Europe and Asia for many years, she added to her wealth of experience in natural healing and holistic development techniques.

Bodo J. Baginski was born on April 10, 1952, as the son of poet Bodo Baginski and author Olli Baginski. After some years of learning, travel, and training, he became a physiotherapist. In 1973, he opened his own practice with a preference for alternative treatments. During his ten years in this profession, he developed a number of patents relating to medical technology. In 1983, his search for further possibilities of holistic healing led him to the Findhorn Community in northern Scotland for one year and later to various Asian countries.

In 1984, Bodo J. Baginski and Shalila Sharamon came together through their common interest in natural, holistic healing. This was followed by a period of lecturing and holding seminars together and the establishment of a book store specializing in esoterica. In 1985, they published their first book, *Reiki - Universal Life Energy*, which received worldwide attention. Further books such as *The Chakra Handbook, Cosmobiological Birth-Control*, and musical guided meditations such as *Chakra Meditation– a Journey into the Energy Centers* (audiotape) and *Chakra Meditation* (double CD) followed. Their inspired works have appeared time and again in the specialized bestseller lists, some of them for several years. Their publications have reached millions of people and have been translated into 20 languages.

In 1990, the two authors retreated to the inspiring stillness of Ireland. They live directly on the Atlantic coast surrounded by unspoiled nature and work on themselves and further books. When they were confronted with the subject of this book, they dedicated a great deal of their time to international research and investigated the promising effects of grapefruit seed extract. Inspired by the results, they interrupted work on three other books without a moment's hesitation in order to put their collected knowledge and experiences onto paper. This is how the present book was created—the first in the world on this subject.

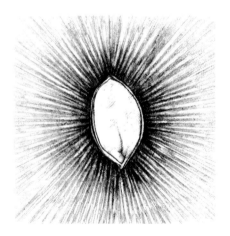

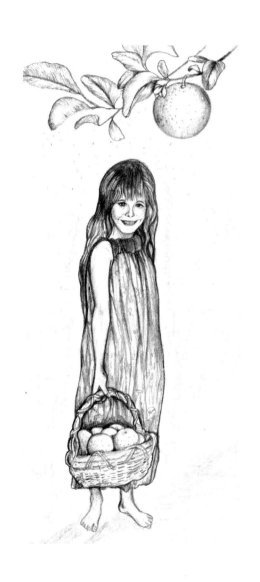

Bibliography

Alternative Medicine Digest: "Grapefruit Seed Extract – A Multipurpose Natural Antibiotic", (Natural Pharmacy), USA, No. 22, 1994

Arndt, Ulrich: "Die Invasion der Pilze – Alarmierende Ergebnisse neuer Blutdiagnose", Esotera, Verlag H. Bauer, Freiburg, Germany, No. 12, 1994

Arndt, Ulrich: "Die Urpilz-Kur – Neue Hoffnung bei vielen Erkrankungen", Esotera, Verlag Hermann Bauer, Freiburg, Germany, No. 1, 1995

Arnoul, Franz: "Der Schlüssel des Lebens", Edition Asklepios, Reichl Verlag, St. Goar, Germany, 3rd. ed., 1995

Béchamp, A.: "Les Mikrozymas", Centre International d´Études A. Béchamp, Paris, 1990

Bioconsultants/Bio-Research Laboratories: "Bacteriocidal Efficacy of Citricidal", Redmond, WA, Dec. 1992

Blechschmidt, Jutta/Meinhof, Wolf: "Candida – Mycosen in der Praxis. Diagnostik und Therapie", Diesbach Verlag, Berlin, 1989

Blecker, Dr. Maria: "Blutuntersuchungen im Dunkelfeld nach Prof. Dr. Günther Enderlein", Semmelweis, Hoya, Germany, 1993

Bolivar, R./Bodey, G. P.: "Candidasis of the Gastrointestinal Tract", Raven Press, New York, 1985

Bursacker, J.: "Epidemiologische Untersuchungen gesunder Rekruten auf Hefepilzbefall von Zunge, Fäzes und Genitale unter besonderer Berücksichtigung zeitsparender Verfahren in der Hefediagnostik", Innaug. Dissertation, Hamburg, 1987

Calori-Domingues, M. A./Fonseca, H.: "Laboratory Evaluation of Chemical Control of Aflatoxin Production in Unshelled Peanuts (Arachis hypogaesa L., with grapefruit seed extract ...)", in: Food Additives and Contaminants 12 (3), Shields, May - June 1995

Cannon: "Teufelskreis – Wenn Antibiotika krank machen", Bircher-Brenner Verlag, Bad Homburg, Germany, issue 1995

Chaitow, Leon: "Candida Albicans: Could Yeast Be Your Problem?", Thorsons, Wellingborough, GB, 1991

Cho, Sung-Hwan et al: "Prevention of Microbial Post-Harvest Injury of Fruits and Vegetables by Using Grapefruit Seed Extract, a Natural Antimicrobial Agent", Journal of the Korean Agricultural Chemical Society, Korea, 36 (4), 265 – 270, 1993

Cho, Sung-Hwan/Seo, Il-Won/Choi, Jong-Duck: "Antimicrobial and Antioxidant Activity of Grapefruit Seed Extract on Fishery Products", Bulletin of the Korean Fisheries Society, Korea, 23 (4), 289 – 296, 1990

Clark, Dr. Hulda Regehr: "The Cure for All Cancers – With 100 Case Histories", ProMotion Publishing, San Diego, CA, 1993

Clark, Dr. Hulda Regehr: "The Cure of All Diseases", ProMotion Publishing, San Diego, CA, 1995

Croog, Dr. med. William G.: "The Yeast Connection", Vintage Books, New York, 2nd. ed., 1986

Croog, Dr. med. William G.: "Candida: Acidophilus and Herbal Remedies, along with an Elimination Diet May Help Sufferers of Chronic Yeast Infections Regain Their Health", Better Nutrition for Today's Living, Vol. 52, No. 5, p. 20, May 1990

Davis, Leonhard J.: "The Natural Health Guide to Children's Health", Natural Health, Vol. 25, No. 6, East West Partners, Nov. 1995

Drury, Susan: "Die Geheimnisse des Teebaums", Windpferd Verlag, Aitrang, Germany, 24th. ed., 1995

Duffus/Slaughler: "Seeds and Their Uses", Wiley, London, 1980

Dumrese, Dr. med. Jost/Haefeli, Bruno: "Handbuch Pleomorphismus. Blutpilze – Blutsymbioten – Blutparasiten ...", Haug Verlag, Heidelberg, 1st. ed., 1995

Dunbar, W. Ph.: "Zur Frage der Stellung der Bakterien, Hefen und Schimmelpilze im System", Semmelweis-Institut, Hoya, Germany, 2nd. ed., 1981

Finck, Hans: "Die Anti-Hefepilz-Diät, Vitalkost gegen Candida albicans", Ehrenwirth Verlag, München, issue 1996

Fiorentin, L. et al: "Growth Inhibition Moulds of the Group Aspergillus Flavus by Grapefruit Seed Extract", Arquivo Brasileiro de Medicina Veterinaria e Zootecnia, 43 (3), 227 – 240, Portugal, 1991

Fonzek, T.: "Pilze auf der Mundschleimhaut und auf Zahnbürsten", Labor Praxis, GIT Verlag, Darmstadt, Germany, No. 4, 1984

Gemeinhardt, H. (Hrsg.): "Endomykosen des Menschen", Fischer Verlag, Stuttgart, Germany, 1989

Ghannoum/Radwan: "Candida Albicans – Candida Adherence to Epithelical Cells", C.R.C. Publications, London, 1990

Ginter, G./Pristautz, H./Beham, H.: "Mykologische Untersuchungen von Speichel und Magensaft bei 100 Endoskopiepatienten", Labormedizin, GIT Verlag, Darmstadt, Germany, No. 6, 1988

Gittlemann, Ann Louise: "Guess What Came To Dinner – Parasites and Your Health", Avery Publishing Group Inc., USA, New York, 1993

Gittlemann, Ann Louise: "The Growing Problem of Parasites", Natural Health, Vol. 23, No. 5, p. 68, East West Partners, Sept. 1993

Goren, R. v./Mendel, K./Balaban, M. (Editors): "Citriculture. Proceedings of the Sixth International Citrus Congress, Middle East", in 4 Vol.s, Margraf Verlag, Weikersheim, Germany, 1989

Gray, Robert: "The Colon Health Handbook", Emerald Publishing, Reno, Nevada, 12th. ed., 1991

Grigoriu/Delacretaz/Barelli: "Lehrbuch der medizinischen Mycologie", Hans Huber Verlag, Stuttgart, Germany, 1994

Guzek, Gaby/Lange, Elisabeth: "Pilze im Körper – Krank ohne Grund", Südwest-Verlag, München, 1995

Häfeli, Bruno: "Die Blut-Mykose", BHS-Labor, Ebikon, 1987

Häfeli, Bruno: "Neues aus der Forschung über die Blut-Mycose", Heft 1 – 4, Verlag BHS-Labor, Pfäffikon/Switzerland

Hauck, Helge: "Candida Mycosen im Alter. Die Bedeutung der Candida albicans-Infektionen der Haut und der Schleimhäute für die Geriatrie", Grosse Verlag, Berlin, 1981

Heideklang, Christine: "Ursachen und Behandlung von Mykosen", Knaur Verlag, München, 1995

Hosch, Harald: "Gesund durch Entsäuerung – Das Säure-Basen-Gleichgewicht wiederherstellen und erhalten", Jopp Verlag, Wiesbaden, Germany, 1994

Ionescu/Kiel/Wichmann-Kunz/Williams/Baum/Levine: "Oral Citrus Seed Extract in Atopic Eczema: In Vitro and In Vivo Studies on Intestinal Microflora", Journal of Orthomolecular Medicine, Vol. 5, No. 3, 1990

Jacobs, Gill: "Candida albicans", Optima Book, Little Brown & Co., London, 4th. ed., 1994

Kimball, H.: "Citrus Processing – Quality Control & Technology", Reinhold van Nost, London, 1991

Kinon, Ulla: "Mycosen – Die (un)heimliche Krankheit", Oesch Verlag, Zürich, 1st. ed., 1986

Kinon, Ulla: "Mycosen", Econ , Düsseldorf, 2nd. ed., 1995

Kinon, Ursula: "Mycosen – Pilzinfektionen der Haut und der inneren Organe", Weltbild , Augsburg, Germany, 1st. ed., 1990

Kinon, Ulla: "Virusinfekte", Verlagsgemeinschaft für Naturheilkunde & Psychologie, Eschborn, 1st. ed., 1989

Kinon, Ulla: "?Allergie? – !Allergie!", Verlagsgemeinschaft für Naturheilkunde & Psychologie, Eschborn, Germany, 3rd. ed., 1995

Klaus, Erna: "Was ist bloß los mit mir? Candida-albicans – Maskierte Pilzerkrankungen", Verlag Rasch und Röhring, Hamburg, 1995

Kreger-van Rij, N. J. W.: "The Yeasts. A Taxonomic Study", Elsevier Service Publishers B.V., Amsterdam, 3rd. ed., 1984

Krehl, P.: "Citrus in Health and Disease", University Press of Florida, 1989

Kroeger, Dr. Hanna: "Parasites – The Enemy Within", Hanna Kroeger Publications, Boulder, Colorado, 1991

Kushner-Resnice, Susan: "Grapefruit Seed Extract – Natural Antibiotic", East-West – Nat. Health Magazine, P. 37 – 39, Jan/Feb. 1992

Lewith, Dr. George T.: "Candida and Thrush", BioMed Publications Ltd, Birmingham, GB, 1990

Lorenzani: "Candida Albicans – Twentieth Century Disease", Keals Publication Inc., London, 1989

Los Angeles Times: "Nature's Way Citronex Supplement Capsules" (contain 130 mg grapefruit seed extract), 11. March, Page 4, The Times Mirror Company, 1992

Malicke, H.: "Langzeitstudie über die Rezedivhäufigkeit der Genitalmykose bei Frauen nach einfacher Lokalbehandlung des Genitals und nach zusätzlicher Lokalbehandlung des Magen-Darm-Traktes", Notabene Medici – Journal für Ärzte, Notamed Verlag, Bad Homburg, Germany, No. 10, 1980

Markus, Dr. med. Harold H./Finck, Hans: "Candida, der entfesselte Hefepilz", Ehrenwirt Verlag, München, 1st. ed., 1995

Markus, Dr. med. Harold H./Finck, Hans: "Ich fühle mich krank und weiß nicht warum – Candida albicans – die maskierte Krankheit.", Ehrenwirt, München, 12th. ed., 1994

Mehlhorn, Heinz (Hrsg.): "Parasitology in Focus – Facts and Trends", Springer Verlag, Berlin, 1988

Meinhof, W.: "Differentialdiagnose Mykose-Ekzem", Der Hautarzt, Springer Verlag, Berlin, No. 26, 1975

Meinhof, W.: "Die intestinale Besiedlung mit Candida albicans und ihre Auswirkung auf einige chronisch-entzündliche Dermatosen", Der Hautarzt, Springer Verlag, Berlin, No. 8, 1995

Mendling, Werner: "Vulvovaginal Candidosis – Theory and Practice", Springer Verlag, Berlin, 1988

Monselise, S. P.: "Citrusfrüchte als Rohware für die Herstellung von Säften und anderen Erzeugnissen", Hempel, Wolfsburg, Germany, 1973

Müller, J.: "Pilze im Gastrointestinaltrakt", Fortschritte der Medizin, Urban und Vogel, München, No. 20, 1982

Müller, J.: "Mikrobiologische Diagnostik und Therapie-kontrolle bei Sproßpilzmykosen", in: "Systemische Mykosen", Editiones Roche, Basel, Switzerland, 1983

Müller-Mees, Elke: "Pilzerkrankungen – Diagnose, Erscheinungsbild und natürliche Behandlung", Knaur Verlag, München, 1995

Nolting, S.: "Die Bedeutung der Candida-Vulvo-Vaginitis und Balnitis unter spezieller Berücksichtigung der Partnerbehandlung", Münchener Medizinische Wochenschrift, MMV Medizin Verlag, München, No. 118, 1976

Nolting, S./Fegeler K.: "Medizinische Mykologie", Springer, Berlin, 1992

Odds, F. C.: "Candida and Candidosis", Baillière Tindall, London, 1988

Olson, Cynthia: "Die Teebaumöl-Hausapotheke", Windpferd Verlag, Aitrang, Germany, 21st. ed., 1995

Parrish, Michael: "Just Call Him The Green Marketeer" (Greenway markets line based on grapefruit seed extract), Los Angeles Times, P. 1, 18th. of Sept. 1993

Patterson, Barbara: "The Allergy Connection", Thorsons, Wellingborough, GB, 1995

Park, S. W./Jeon, J. H./Kim, H. S./Joung, H. : "Effect of Grapefruit Seed Extract on Penicillium Growth and Tuberization in Tissue Culture of Potato (Solanum Tuberosum L.)", Hauguk Wonye Hakoe Chi, Korea, v. 36 (2) 1995/Journal of the Korean Society for Horticultural Science, Korea, 36 (2), P. 179 – 184, 1995

Prasad, Rajendra: "Candida Albicans – Cellular and Molecular Biology", Springer Verlag, Berlin, 1991

Prigge, W./Prigge-Stein, R.: "Nativblutuntersuchungen im Dunkelfeld und bioelektronische Messung nach Vincent – Arbeitsmappe III", Selbstverlag, Hannover, Germany, 1990

Pschyrembel, Prof. Dr. Dr. Willibald: "Klinisches Wörterbuch", Verlag de Gruyter, Berlin, 257th. ed., 1993

Pulverer, Gerhard: "Medizinische Mikrobiologie und Parasitologie für Krankenpflegeberufe", Thieme, Stuttgart, Germany, 2nd. ed., 1988

Ranzani, M.R./Fonseca, H.: "Mycological Evaluation of Chemically-Treated Unshelled Peanuts (with Grapefruit Seed Extrakt ...)", Food Additives and Contaminants, 12 (3), Shields, May-June 1995

Reinhold, Horst G.: "Citruswirtschaft in Israel. Eine geographische Untersuchung des Agrumenbau, seiner Voraussetzungen, Formen und Möglichkeiten", Geographisches Institut der Universität Heidelberg, Heidelberg, Germany, 1975

Rieth, H.: "Pathologische Gärung im Darm durch pathogene Hefen", Pilzdialog – Praktische Mykologie, Schwarzeck Verlag, Ottobrunn, Germany, No. 1, 1984

Rieth, H.: "Das Recht auf Pilz-freie Geburt", Pilzdialog – Praktische Mykologie, Schwarzeck Verlag, Ottobrunn, Germany, No. 2, 1984

Rieth, H.: "Anti-Pilz-Diät gegen pathogene Hefen im Intestinaltrakt", Pilzdialog/Praktische Mykologie, Schwarzeck, Ottobrunn, Germany, No. 3, 1985

Rieth, H.: "Mykosen – Anti-Pilz-Diät", Notamed, Melsungen, Germany, 1988

Rippere, Vickey: "The Allergy Problem", Thornsons, Wellingborough, GB, 1989

Rochlitz, Dr. med. Steven: "Allergies and Candida", Human Ecology Balancing Sciences Inc., New York, 1988

Sachs, Dr. med. Allan: "Grapefruit Seed Extract – A Revolution in Germ Control", To Your Health Magazine, USA, issue April/May 1993

Sachs, Dr. med. Allan: "Grapefruit Seed Extract – The Swiss Army Knife of Germ Control", Health Store News, USA, issue Aug./Sept. 1993

Saltarelli: "Candida Albicans – The Pathogenic Lungs", Hemisphere Publication, USA, 1989

Schepper: "Candida Albicans – Diet Against It", Foulsham Pub., GB, 1989

Schneider, Dr. med. Ernst: "Die grossen 5 der Heilkraft" – 5 volumes, Edited by: Deutscher Verein für Gesundheitspflege, Vol. I "Nutze die Heilkraft unserer Nahrung – Geleitwort von Ralph Bircher", Saatkorn Verlag, Hamburg, 5th. ed., 1989

Schütz, B.: "Hefepilze. Ein Kompendium hefebedingter Erkrankungen", Institut für Mikroökologie, Herborn, Germany, 1994

Schütz, B./Keiner, K./Zimmermann, K.: "Candida-Mykosen", Erfahrungsheilkunde – Acta medica empirica – Zeitschrift für die ärztliche Praxis, Haug Verlag, Heidelberg, Germany, No. 9, 1994

Schwerdtle, Dr. Cornelia/Arnoul, Franz: "Einführung in die Dunkelfelddiagnostik", Semmelweis Verlag, Hoya, Germany, 1st. ed., 1993

Sichel/Sichel: "Relief From Candida – Allergies and Ill Health", S. Millner Publications, Australia, 1990

Skolnick, Dr. Mitchell: "Grapefruit Seed Extract", The Trend Journal, Vol. I, No. 1, Pg. 3, The Trends Research Institute, USA, Winter Report 1992

Tantaoui-Elaraki, A. et al: "Inhibition of the Garden Cress Seed (and Grapefruit Seed Extract) Germination by Penicillium Italicum Wehmer and Penicillium Digitatum (Pers. Ex. Fr.) Sacch. Culture Filtrates", 25 (4), P. 353 – 356, Lebensmittel-Wissenschaft & Technologie, Academic Press Inc., London, 1992

The Third Opinion: "Botanical Extract Stops Diarrhea, Strep Throat, Gingivitis, Candidiasis, and More ..." – "A Revolutionary New Antiviral Agent!" – "University Of Georgia Evaluates Citrus Extract" – "Intestinal Candidiasis Stopped With Grapefruit Seed Extract" – "Hospitals Use Citrus Extract ... Environmentally Safe and Non-Toxic" – "Chlorine-Free Jacuzzi" – "Citrus Extract Replaces Chlorine As Wastewater Effluent Treatment" – "First Aid For Drinking Water" – "Soil Test Confirmation: Citrus Extract Is Environmentally Safe", (Magazine – For the Health & Environmentally Conscious Professional) Pentaluma, CA, Vol. I & II, 1994

Trickett, Shirley: "Coping with Candida", Sheldon Press, London, 1994

Trickett, Shirley: "Candida Albicans – Over 100 Yeast-Free and Sugar-Free Recipes", Thorsons, London, 1995

Trowbridge, J. P./Walker, M.: "The Yeast Syndrome", Bantam, New York, 1986

Truss, Dr. med. C. Orion: "The Missing Diagnosis", Birmingham, GB, 1982

Tumbay, Ed.: "Candida Albicans and Candidamycosis – Symposium Proceedings", Plenum Publications Co., London, 1991

Turner/Simonsen: "Candida Albicans – Special Diet Cookbook", Thorsons, Wellingborough, 1989

Vasey, Christopher: "Die Entgiftung des Körpers", Midena Verlag, Augsburg, Germany, 1994

Villequez, E.: "Der latente Parasitismus der Blutzellen beim Menschen, besonders im Blut der Krebskranken", Semmelweis-Institut, Hoya, Germany, 1956

Vucovic, Laurel: "Treating Common Health Problems Naturally; Consumer Guide to Women´s Health" (suggests grapefruit seed extract), Natural Health, Vol. 24, No. 4, P. 86, East West Partners, USA, July 1994

Weinberger, Stanley: "Parasites – An Epidemic in Disguise", Healing Within Products, Larkspur, California, 2nd. ed., 1994

Weise, Dr. D. O.: "Harmonische Ernährung. Wie Sie bewußter werden und Ihre persönliche gesunde Ernährung intuitiv selbst finden", Smaragdina Verlag, München, 1st. ed., 1990

Wetzel, W. E./Sziegoleit, A./Weckler, C.: "Karies-Candidose des Milchgebisses bei Kleinkindern", Labormedizin, GIT Verlag, Darmstadt, Germany, 3rd. ed., 1983

White, Linda B.: "Bumps, Bruises and Bites: Basic First Aid for The Whole Family" (includes grapefruit seed extract), Mothering, No. 74, P. 46, Peggy O´Mara, USA, March 1995

Wiedemann, Dr. med. Michael: "Der Gesundheit auf der Spur – Die Mikro-Nährstoffe der Orthomolekularmedizin", Ariston Verlag, Geneva, Switzerland, 1994

Winner, H. I./Hurly, R.: "Symposium on Candida Infections", Livingstone Pub., Edinburgh, GB, 1966

Wright, Brian/Wright, Celia: "Grapefruit Seed Extrakt – A Natural Antibiotic", Beyond Nutrition (Magazine), Burwash Common, East Sussex, GB, Autumn 1994

Wright, Brian/Wright, Celia: "The Helicobacter Story" – "Readers Report – Grapefruit Seed Experiment", Beyond Nutrition (Magazine), Burwash Common, East Sussex, GB, Spring 1995

Scientific Analyses, Studies and Laboratory Tests*

BC Research - British Columbia Research Corp.,Vancouver, B.C., Canada: "Final Report Bacteriocidal Efficacy of Citricidal", Client: EcoTrend, North Vancouver, B.C., Canada, Completion: March 1992

Bio/Chem Research Inc., Lakeport, CA, USA: "Citricidal – Mechanism of Action and Evaluation as a Disinfectant", Client: Bio/Chem Research Inc., Lakeport, CA, USA. Own study. Completion: not stated

Bio Research Laboratories Inc., Redmond, WA, USA: "Bacteriocidal Efficacy of Citricidal – Laboratory Report", Client: Mr. John Harrison, EcoTrend, North Vancouver, B.C., Canada, Completion: December 9, 1992

Bio Research Laboratories Inc., Redmond, WA, USA: "Biodegradability of Citricidal Liquid – Laboratory Report", Client: Mr. Richard Perry, Bio/Chem Research Inc., Lakeport, CA, USA, Completion: August 31, 1994

Brigham Young University, Provo, UT, USA: "Evaluation Report of the Inhibitory Properties of Citricidal® / Inhibition of Bacteria and Yeast by Citricidal®", Client: Bio/Chem Research Inc., Lakeport, CA, USA, Completion: September 20, 1990

Great Smokies Diagnostic Laboratory, Asheville, N.C., USA: "Citricidal®-Bacterial and Yeast Sensitivity Tests", Client: Bio/Chem Research Inc., Lakeport, CA, USA, Completion: July 1991

Institut Pasteur, Paris, Frankreich: "In Vitro Study of the Inactivation of HIV by Citricidal®", Client: Bio/Chem Research, Lakeport, CA, USA, (there have only been partial results available up to now. The study was not completely finished yet, at the time of printing of this book in 1996)

Northview Pacific Laboratories Inc., Berkeley, CA, USA: "Test Article Identification: Citricidal, 0,2 %. Test Performed: USP Preservative Effectiveness Test", Client: Mr. Richard Perry, Bio/Chem Research Inc., Lakeport, CA, USA, Completion: June 8, 1995

Northview Pacific Laboratories Inc., Berkeley, CA, USA: "Test Article Identification: Methylparaben, 0,2 %. Test Performed: USP Preservative Challenge Test", Client: Mr. Richard Perry, Bio/

---

* Existing documentation on the effect of grapefruit seed extract that was available for evaluation to the authors for the work of this book.

Chem Research Inc., Lakeport, CA, USA, Completion: June 8, 1995

Northview Pacific Laboratories Inc., Berkeley, CA, USA: "Citricidal Test: Acute Oral Toxicity", Client: Mr. Kenneth Stryker, Matsuhitu Chemical Corp., Carson City, NV, USA, Completion: July 6, 1995

Southern Research Institute, USA: "Test Comparing the Antiviral, Antibacterial & Antifungal Properties of a New Disinfectant Formulation (ImuSol) Containing 500 ppm Citricidal® with Commercially Available Disinfectant Nolvasan", Client: ImuTech Inc., Huntington Valley, PA, USA, Completion: November 26, 1984

United States Department of Agriculture, Greenport, New York, USA: "Citricidal® Effective Against Three Animal Viruses: Foot-and-Mouth Disease (FMD), African Swine Fever (ASF), Swine Vesicular Disease (SVD)", Client: Dr. Jacob Harich, Lakeport, CA, USA, Completion: September 7, 1982

United States Department of Agriculture, Hyattsville, MD, USA: "The Effect of Citricidal Against Avian Influenza", Client: Dr. Jacob Harich, Lakeport, CA, USA, Completion: May 7, 1984

University of Georgia / College of Agriculture, Department of Poultry Science, Athens, Georgia, USA: "Inhibitory Effect of Citricidal® Against Lysteria Monocytogenes", Client: Bio/Chem Research Inc., Lakeport, CA, USA, Completion: 24th. of February 1984

University of Georgia / College of Agriculture, Department of Poultry Science, Athens, Georgia, USA: "Citricidal® as a Feed Preservative, Mold Inhibitor, Antioxidant and for Use with Fish", Client: Bio/Chem Research Inc., Lakeport, CA, USA, Completion: not stated

Valley Microbiology Services, Palo Alto, CA, USA: "Citricidal® Inhibition of Growth of Campylobacter Jejuni and Helicobacter Pylori", Client: Bio/Chem Research Inc., Lakeport, CA, USA, Completion: July 11, 1991

Valley Microbiology Services, Palo Alto, CA, USA: "Citricidal® Skin Cleanser Inhibition of Growth of Escherichia Coli, Salmonella Typhimurium and Staphylococcus Aureus", Client: Bio/Chem Research Inc., Lakeport, CA, USA, Completion: July 11, 1991

Valley Microbiology Services, Palo Alto, CA, USA: "Citricidal® Inhibition of Growth of Shigella Dysenteriae", Client: Bio/Chem Research Inc., Lakeport, CA, USA, Completion: September 9, 1991

Valley Microbiology Services, Palo Alto, CA, USA: "Citricidal® Inhibition of Growth of Chlamydia Trachomatis", Client: Bio/

Chem Research Inc., Lakeport, CA, USA, Completion: September 20, 1991

Valley Microbiology Services, Palo Alto, CA, USA: "Citricidal® Inhibition of Growth of Vibrio Cholerae", Client: Bio/Chem Research Inc., Lakeport, CA, USA, Completion: November 19, 1991

Valley Microbiology Services, Palo Alto, CA, USA: "Citricidal® Determination of Inhibition of Giardia Lamblia", Client: Bio/ Chem Research Inc., Lakeport, CA, USA, Completion: November 26, 1991

Valley Microbiology Services, Palo Alto, CA, USA: "Inhibitory Effects of Citricidal® Against Legionella Pneumophila", Client: Bio/Chem Research Inc., Lakeport, CA, USA, Completion: not stated

Valley Microbiology Services, Palo Alto, CA, USA: "Citricidal® – Two-fold Serial Dilution Tests on Bacteria and Fungi", Client: Bio/Chem Research Inc., Lakeport, CA, USA, Completion: not stated

Valley Microbiology Services, Palo Alto, CA, USA: "Salmonella Trial Evaluation of the Effect of Citricidal on Chicken Carcasses (in Reducing Salmonella Typhimurium)", Client: Bio/Chem Research Inc., Lakeport, CA, USA, Completion: not stated

In addition, the authors had available to some extent the internal research documentation, laboratory analyses, and study results from the following companies:

BIO/CHEM Research Inc., Lakeport, CA, USA
ECOTREND Products Ltd., North Vancouver, BC, Canada
HELIOS MOLLE KONSORTIENT – DANSK HELIOS, Frederica, Denmark
HIGHER NATURE, Burwash Common, East Sussex, GB
IMHOTEP Inc., Ruby, NY, USA
MEDAFARM AG, Münchenstein, Switzerland
NUTRIBIOTIC Inc., Lakeport, CA, USA
GSE-Vertrieb, Saarbrücken, Germany
PHYTOMED IRELAND Ltd., Dublin, Ireland
PRIMAVERA LIFE GmbH, Sulzberg, Germany

in addition to the research results of a number of private researches from four countries.

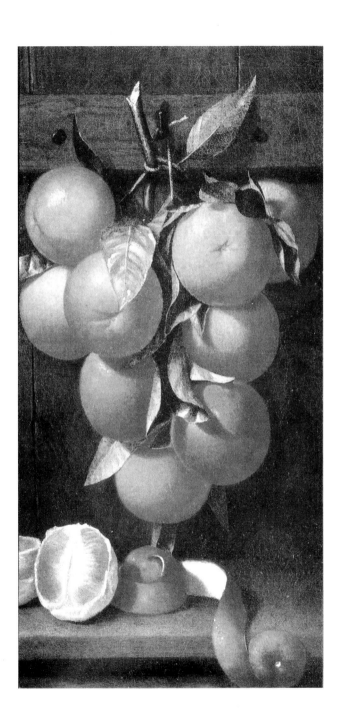

Index

B

139

lip blisters 74
lips 25
Listeria monocytogenes 106
liver 43, 44, 50, 51, 55
  fluke 55
livestock 61, 88
Loefflerella
  mallei 107
  pseudomallei 107
lovage 90
love 40
lungs 50, 55, 58, 82, 102
lymphatic system 49, 54
lymphogranuloma 55
Lynn, Dr. C. W. 63

M

Malaysia 15
male disorders 50
malnutrition 54
Malt lymphoma 48
mammals 85
manufacturers 18, 21, 72 - 74, 80, 103, 109, 117, 152
marjoram 90
Marshall, Barry 48
mastitis 19
measles virus, *Morbillium* 109
meat 20, 50, 78, 80, 88, 89
medical equipment 21
medication 57, 59
medicine chest 30
Mediterranean 103
memory 50, 54
Mendall, Dr. 48
meningitis 50
mental 40, 41
mercury amalgam
  teeth 40
metabolic
  processes 26
  products 26, 40, 55
Mexico 8, 12, 15, 19, 63
mice 101
micro-organisms 59
microspore 67
midges 93
midwives 76, 117
migraine 50, 58

milking machinery 91
Mold 50
  fruit 80
  walls 52
mold 17, 20, 49, 50, 52, 78, 93, 104, 109
  fruit 78
  inhibitor 20
  seeds 97
  snow 94
  soil 78
Molecular Weight 104
Monilia albicans 108
Moraxella
  duplex 107
  glucidolytica 107
Morbillium 109
Morocco 12
mouth 18, 24, 66, 74, 75
  ulcer 24, 66
  vetinary 87
  wash 24, 71
Mucor 49
mucous membranes 23, 35, 50, 71
muscle 55, 58
Mycobacterium
  phelei 106
  smegmatis 106
  tuberculosis 106
mycosis 49
Mycosis Pedis 32

N

nail 18, 33, 34, 68, 71, 83
  bed 34
  file 34
naringenin rutinosid 13, 99
naringin 12, 13, 99
nasal rinse 27
nasal spray 27
naturopaths 49, 76, 117
naturopathy 39
nausea 46
Neisseria catarrhalis 107
neohesperidin 13, 99
nerves 51
nettle 90
nettle rash 31
neurosis 58

U

ulcer 50, 55
  duodenal 48
  gastric 47
  leg 31, 68
  mouth 24
  nasal 27
underarm odor 71
underwear 35, 37
Universidad Automóma de Nuevo 15
University of
  Arkansas 15
  Georgia 15
  Malaya 15
  Ricardo Palma 15
  San Marcos 15, 20
  Sao Paulo 15, 21
  Virginia 55
urethra 36, 37
urethritis 36
urine
  blood 66
US Department of Agriculture 15, 89
US Department of Health 18
USA 8, 12, 15, 16, 21, 22, 54 - 56, 72,
  82, 101 - 105, 109, 121
uterus 55
UV rays 82

V

vaccinations 20, 62
vagina 35, 67, 68
  hygiene 36
  infection 36
vaginal
  Candida 19, 35
  discharge 36
  flora 35
  infections 18
  rinse 35
vaginitis 35, 61
Valley Microbiology Services 105
varnishes 55
vegetables 20, 50, 52, 78, 80, 103
vermifuges 20, 56, 85, 88
vet 19, 84, 90
Vibrio
  cholerae 46, 108

eltor 108
viral
  cultures 99
  infection 39, 46
virus 16, 43, 49, 55, 61, 119
  cosmetics 74
  domestic 77
  external 23
  flu 45, 109
  herpes 24, 25, 109
  HIV 19, 55
  internal 39
  measles 109
  test results 105
  vetinary 86, 91, 92
    ASF 89
    MKS 89
viscosity 104
vitamin
  B1 12
  C 12
  P 13
voice 70
vomiting 46

W

Warren, Robert 47, 48
warts 32
Water
  tap 42
water
  chlorinated 22
  cholera 46
  cleaning 83, 90
  drinking 22, 63, 64, 83, 84, 103
    contaminated 47, 56, 84
    treatment 84
    vetinary 87, 88, 89
  fish 20
  pure 42
  retention 58
  sewage 22
  washing 35, 36
  waste 83
  well 84
water pik 25, 26, 71
well 84
wheat 95
whirlpool 22, 82

Addresses and Supply Sources

Because of the continuously expanding range of products in relation to grapefruit seed extract articles, Lotus Light offers a free information service.

On request, you can receive the current European list of information with corresponding product information, addresses of manufacturers, suppliers, and distributors. It also contains European addresses of institutes that perform the blood test described in this book. As U.S.A. sources become known they will be added to this listing.

For this information, write to:

Lotus Light Publications
"Grapefruit Seed Extract"
P.O. Box 325
Twin Lakes, WI 53181
USA

Please enclose a large self-addressed and stamped envelope with your letter.

For U.S.A. inquiries, the following distributors supply Grapefruit Seed Extract products or can advise you of sources:

WHOLESALE
Contact with your business name,
resale number or practioner license.

LOTUS LIGHT ENTERPRISES, INC.
Box 1008 GS
Silver Lake, WI 53170
Voice 414/889-8501 • Fax 414/889-8591

RETAIL
INTERNATURAL
33719 116th Street Box GS
Twin Lakes, WI 53181

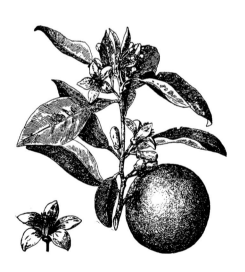